Sexual Dysfunction

Advances in Psychosomatic Medicine

Vol. 29

Series Editor

T.N. Wise Falls Church, Va.

Editors

G.A. Fava Bologna

I. Fukunishi Tokyo

M.B. Rosenthal Cleveland, Ohio

Sexual Dysfunction

The Brain-Body Connection

Volume Editor

R. Balon Detroit, Mich.

5 figures and 4 tables, 2008

KARGER Basel · Freiburg · Paris · London · New York · Bangalore · Bangkok · Shanghai · Singapore · Tokyo · Sydney

Advances in Psychosomatic Medicine

Founded 1960 by
F. Deutsch (Cambridge, Mass.)
A. Jores (Hamburg)
B. Stockvis (Leiden)

Continued 1972–1982 by
F. Reichsman (Brooklyn, N.Y.)

Library of Congress Cataloging-in-Publication Data

Sexual dysfunction : the brain-body connection/ volume editor, R. Balon.
p. ; cm. – (Advances in psychosomatic medicine, ISSN 0065-3268 ; v. 29)
Includes bibliographical references and index.
ISBN 978-3-8055-8357-2 (hard cover: alk. paper)
1. Sexual disorders. I. Balon, Richard. II. Series.
[DNLM: 1. Sexual Dysfunction, Physiological. 2. Sexual Dysfunctions, Psychological. W1 AD81 v.29 2008 / WJ 709 S5183 2008]
RC556.S478 2008
616.85′83–dc22 2008009250

Bibliographic Indices. This publication is listed in bibliographic services, including Current Contents® PubMed/MEDLINE

Drug Dosage. The authors and the publisher have exerted every effort to ensure that drug selection and dosage set forth in this text are in accord with current recommendations and practice at the time of publication. However, in view of ongoing research, changes in government regulations, and the constant flow of information relating to drug therapy and drug reactions, the reader is urged to check the package insert for each drug for any change in indications and dosage and for added warnings and precautions. This is particularly important when the recommended agent is a new and/or infrequently employed drug.

www.karger.com
Printed in Switzerland on acid-free and non-aging paper (ISO 9706) by Reinhardt Druck, Basel
ISSN 0065–3268
ISBN 978–3–8055–8357–2

Contents

Balon R (ed): Sexual Dysfunction. The Brain-Body Connection.
Adv Psychosom Med. Basel, Karger, 2008, vol 29, pp 1–6

Introduction: New Developments in the Area of Sexual Dysfunction(s)

Richard Balon

Department of Psychiatry and Behavioral Neurosciences,
Wayne State University School of Medicine, Detroit, Mich., USA

Abstract

New developments in the area of sexual dysfunction, e.g. epidemiology and pharmacological treatment, are reviewed. Areas where new developments/changes are needed, such as diagnosis of sexual dysfunction and research methodology, are also briefly discussed.

Sex, together with eating and sleeping, is one of the basic drives. Impairment of this drive/sexual functioning can have a profound impact on the person's quality of life and other aspects of functioning. Sexual behavior represents a very complex and interesting interaction of biology and psychology. Even an ostensibly simple phenomenon such as erection represents a complex interaction of the central and peripheral nervous systems modified by various psychological factors, and impacted by factors such as vascular abnormalities, various physical illnesses, aging, substance abuse and many others. Including among them, as Goldstein noted in his aptly named editorial 'In the end, "sex is complicated"' [1], is the fact that, 'sexual function and dysfunction involve the couple, which does not make sex any less complicated'. Goldstein [1] also correctly notes that we know very little about sex. It is actually surprising how little we really know, in spite of the fact that sex is an important and popular part of our life, culture, arts, ordinary talks and even everyday conversations and jokes.

The general public seems to agree that sex is an important part of their life and that sexual health is important for peoples' overall well-being. In a U.S. poll discussed by Marwick [2], among married men, 91% ranked a satisfying sex life as important, as did 84% of married women. In addition, '94% of those polled said that sexual enjoyment added to the quality of life at any age, while half said that sexual problems should not be accepted as a consequence of aging'. More than 90% of those polled in this unscientific survey also believed that unsatisfactory sex life can cause numerous other problems such as depression or breakup of marriage. The popular belief of the importance of sexual well-being has been also confirmed in various scientific studies. For instance, Laumann et al. [3] found that subjective sexual well-being was correlated with overall happiness in both men and women in various countries.

Results of epidemiological studies suggest that impairment of sexual function, i.e. sexual dysfunction, is definitely quite frequent, and that is an important health concern [4]. According to a well-publicized U.S. study of Laumann et al. [4], sexual dysfunction is fairly prevalent in women (43%) as well as men (31%). These authors also observed that the experience of sexual dysfunction is more likely among women and men with poor physical and emotional health, and that sexual dysfunction is highly associated with negative experiences in sexual relationships and overall well-being [4]. An international study [5] yielded similar prevalence rates. For instance, lack of interest in sex and inability to reach orgasm were the most common sexual problems in women across world regions, ranging from 26 to 43%, and 18 to 41%, respectively. Interestingly, in most cases, the reported prevalence of sexual problems was higher in East Asia and Southeast Asia than in other regions of the world [5]. In spite of many methodological problems of this (e.g. low response rate, differences in recruitments of samples) and other studies (e.g. diagnostic criteria not rigorous enough), the results strongly suggest that sexual dysfunction(s) is a frequent problem throughout the world, and that there is a relatively unambiguous relationship between the frequency of dysfunction and age in both men and women [6]. Yet, I would suggest that the overall nonindustry-sponsored spending on research in this area is probably significantly less than in many areas of medicine and mental health.

Nevertheless, we have been witnessing enormous developments in the study of human sexuality during the last few decades. This area has become multidisciplinary, with urology, obstetrics and gynecology, sexology, psychology and basic sciences stepping up their efforts and interests. A new 'discipline', sexual medicine, seems to be emerging. Interestingly, the field of psychiatry appears to be less and less involved and interested in the area of human sexuality and sexual dysfunction. This trend is quite unfortunate, especially since psychiatry and neurosciences are at the crossroads of many of these disciplines and seem to be uniquely qualified and fitted to synthesize the findings from the medical and psychological disciplines.

What Are the Areas of Rapid Development and Areas/Issues That Are in Need of Development?

Treatment

The most significant developments over the last two decades have happened in the area of treatment of sexual dysfunction, more specifically treatment of erectile dysfunction and premature ejaculation. The introduction of intraurethral and intracorporeal administration of prostaglandin E-1 for treatment of erectile dysfunction, followed by the accidental discovery of the efficacy of sildenafil, launched a new era of 'sexual pharmacology' [7]. The other two phosphodiesterase-5 inhibitors, tadalafil and vardenafil (both 'me-too' drugs) appeared soon. The phosphodiesterase-5 inhibitors have been tried in various indications in men and women. They have been found effective in erectile dysfunction of various etiologies, and in some male urological difficulties, e.g. lower urinary tract symptoms in men [8]. Since its launch in the United States in 1998, sildenafil has been approved in over 110 countries [9], and over 500 million tablets of sildenafil have been distributed worldwide by 2002 [8]. The number of studies and reports on sildenafil has been enormous – a recent (January 2008) PubMed search of sildenafil and erectile dysfunction yielded a staggering number of 1,778 references, and additional search for tadalafil and vardenafil and erectile dysfunction revealed over 700 additional references. There are more phosphodiesterase-5 inhibitors that may potentially enter the market, such as avanafil, udenafil, mirodenafil and others [10]. Similar to the results of studies of sildenafil in male erectile disorder, but less spectacular and less published, are the results of treatment studies of premature ejaculation [e.g. 11]. Some selective serotonin reuptake inhibitors such as fluoxetine, paroxetine and sertraline, and serotonergic tricyclic antidepressant clomipramine have gradually become the first-line treatment for premature ejaculation.

Unfortunately, advancements in pharmacological treatment of sexual dysfunctions in women have been less than modest. The efficacy of sildenafil was examined in female sexual arousal disorder, too. In spite of some favorable early reports from small trials, the results of large clinical trials [e.g. 12] did not confirm sildenafil's efficacy in this indication, and thus Pfizer ultimately terminated its trials of sildenafil in women. Some studies suggest efficacy of bupropion in hypoactive sexual desire disorder in premenopausal nondepressed women [13], and testosterone in postmenopausal women with hypoactive sexual desire disorder [14]. Maybe the new classes of drugs such as melanocortins [15] will be more successful in treatment of sexual dysfunction in women. The results of some preclinical trials with bremelanotide [16] suggest that this compound may be useful in the treatment of hypoactive sexual desire disorders.

The advances of treatment of sexual dysfunctions have certainly not been limited to the area of pharmacotherapy. An example of the continuous and increasing developments in the area of sex therapy is the fourth edition of Leiblum's *Principles and Practice of Sex Therapy* [17].

Sexual Dysfunction and Somatic Illness

The field of medicine has started to pay more attention to sexuality in connection to other illnesses. As Basson [18] and Basson and Schultz [19] noted, sexual sequelae of chronic somatic illnesses are quite common. Numerous endocrine, neurological, immunological, vascular and other diseases can profoundly negatively affect sexual functioning. However, we clearly need more research in this area, especially with a focus on pathophysiology of sexual dysfunction during various chronic somatic (and mental) illnesses and treatment of sexual dysfunction associated with these illnesses.

Journals, Books

Another area of growth is scientific publications, namely scientific journals and books devoted to the topic of sexuality. The field of journals has been gradually expanding and we now have several older and newer journals devoted to sexuality and sexual dysfunction available, such as *The Journal of Sex and Marital Therapy, The Journal of Sexual Medicine, Archives of Sexual Behavior, Journal of Sex Research*, and *International Journal of Impotence Research*. Journals focused on human sexuality are published also in non-English-speaking countries. One such example is *Sexuologia (Sexology)* published by the Slovak Society for Sexology.

Numerous books focusing on various aspects of human sexuality have been published lately; examples include the mentioned volumes on sex therapy [17], and sexual pharmacology [7], or the *Handbook of Clinical Sexuality for Mental Health Professionals* [20] and *Handbook of Sexual Dysfunction* [21].

Organizations

Another sign of the increased interest in human sexuality is the growing number of professional societies in this field. Examples of these societies include:

1 The International Society for Sexual Medicine (secretariat@ISSM.info), which includes several regional organizations: (a) Africa Gulf Society for Sexual Medicine; (b) Asia Pacific Society for Sexual Medicine (www.apssm.org); (c) European Society for Sexual Medicine (http://www.essm.org); (d) Latin American Society for Sexual Medicine – Sociedad Latinoamericana de Medicina Sexual (www.SLAMSnet.org); (e) Sexual Medicine Society of North America (www. amsna.org)
2 International Society for the Study of Women's Sexual Health (info@isswsh.org)
3 International Academy of Sex Research (www.iasr.org)

Many countries have their own national organizations in the area of human sexuality. Examples include the Dutch Society for Sexology, Danish Association for Clinical Sexology (Dansk Forening for Klinisk Sexologi), Nordic Association for Clinical Sexology, German Society for Social-Scientific Sexuality Research, Indonesian Association for Sexology, Slovak Society for Sexology, and four organizations in North America: The Society of the Scientific Study of Sexuality, The American Association of Sex Educators, Counselors, and Therapists, The Society for Sex Therapy and Research, and The Sexuality Information and Education Council of the United States.

Areas That Need More Attention and Development – Diagnosis and Research Methodology

Diagnosis

The diagnostic criteria of sexual dysfunction(s) remain one of the significant weaknesses of sexology or sexual medicine. Our nosology is of poor quality [6] and quite imprecise. We are not clear on when a sexual problem becomes a sexual dysfunction [22]. We have discussed diagnostic issues [23, 24] that need to be addressed in the future discussions of the criteria of sexual dysfunction(s), such as the need for a specific duration criterion of sexual dysfunction, and whether distress should be used as a diagnostic criterion of sexual dysfunction. Further nosology/classification issues raise questions of including new diagnostic entities (e.g. persistent genital arousal disorder in women), reclassifying dyspareunia, possibly deleting sexual aversion disorder and a host of other issues [24], such as whether to classify asexuality as a sexual dysfunction [25]. The existing diagnostic criteria are definitely far from being ideal, and that certainly hinders our research and clinical practice.

Research Methodology

DeRogatis and Burnett [26] summarized some of the key methodological issues in sexual medicine research. The lack of a meaningful diagnostic system is certainly a major problem. The next very important issue is the lack of a good, widely accepted set of outcome measures. We clearly have too many scales and questionnaires, some poorly validated, some measuring too little or too much. As DeRogatis and Burnett [26] pointed out, no single measure appears clearly superior to the others. Most, if not all our studies also lack explicitly defined research populations [26]. We also need to be more precise in our definitions and taxonomy – DeRogatis and Burnett [26] suggest that we 'can no longer afford the luxury of taxonomic imprecision, which has allowed us to treat terms like "sexual desire", "sexual interest", and "sexual motivation" as synonyms for an identical state. They are not. They refer to distinct, albeit overlapping, entities, a distinction which must be reflected in our clinical science'. Last but not least, we need to develop better methods to measure clinical (vs. statistical) significance in our treatment studies.

Afterword

This volume of *Advances in Psychosomatic Medicine* presents some of the discussed new developments in the area of sexual dysfunction such as research-oriented evaluation, treatment of some of the sexual dysfunctions, the intertwining of sexual dysfunction with mental and physical illness, with substance abuse and with psychotropic medications, and last but not least, news from the area of imaging.

It is obvious that the area of human sexuality in general, and sexual dysfunction in particular, has been undergoing enormous development and advances. Hopefully, this volume will help interested readers sort out some of the newest developments and become more interested/involved in this area.

References

1 Goldstein I: Editorial. In the end, 'sex is complicated'. J Sex Med 2007;4:523–525.
2 Marwick C: Survey says patients expect little physician help on sex. JAMA 1999;281:2173–2174.
3 Laumann EO, Paik A, Glasser DB, Kang J-H, Wang T, Levinson B, Moreira ED, Nicolosi A, Gingell C: A cross-national study of subjective well-being among older women and men: findings from the Global Study of Sexual Attitudes and Behaviors. Arch Sex Behav 2006; 35:145–161.
4 Laumann EO, Paik A, Rosen RC: Sexual dysfunction in the United States. JAMA 1999;281:537–544.
5 Laumann EO, Nicolosi A, Glasser DB, Paik A, Gingell C, Moreira E, Wang T, for the GSSAB Investigators' Group: Sexual problems among women and men aged 40–80 years: prevalence and correlates identified in the Global Study of Sexual Attitudes and Behaviors. Int J Impot Res 2005;17:39–57.
6 DeRogatis LR, Burnett AL: The epidemiology of sexual dysfunction. J Sex Med 2008;5:289–300.
7 Segraves RT, Balon R: Sexual pharmacology. Fast facts. New York, WW Norton, 2003.
8 Gales BJ, Gales MA: Phosphodiesterase-5 inhibitors for lower urinary tract symptoms in men. Ann Pharmacother 2008;42:111–115.
9 Osterloh IH, Riley A: Clinical update on sildenafil citrate. Br J Clin Pharmacol 2002;53:219–223.
10 Hatzimouratidis K, Hatzichristou DG: Looking to the future for erectile dysfunction therapies. Drugs 2008;68:231–250.
11 Waldinger MD: Premature ejaculation: definition and drug treatment. Drugs 2007;67:547–568.
12 Basson R, McInness R, Smith MD, Hodgson G, Koppiker N: Efficacy and safety of sildenafil citrate in women with sexual dysfunction associated with female sexual arousal disorder. J Womens Health Gend Based Med 2002;11:367–377.
13 Segraves RT, Clayton A, Croft H, Wolf A, Warnock J: Bupropion sustained release for the treatment of hypoactive sexual desire disorder in premenopausal women. J Clin Psychopharmacol 2004;24:339–342.
14 Kingsberg S, Shifren J, Wekselman K, Rodenberg C, Koochaki P: Evaluation of the clinical relevance of benefits associated with transdermal testosterone treatment in postmenopausal women with hypoactive sexual desire disorder. J Sex Med 2007;4:1001–1008.
15 Shadiack AM, Sharma SD, Earle DC, Spana C, Hallam TJ: Melanocortins in the treatment of male and female sexual dysfunction. Curr Top Med Chem 2007;7:137–144.
16 Pfaus J, Giuliano F, Gelez H: Bremelanotide: an overview of preclinical CNS effects on female sexual dysfunction. J Sex Med 2007;4(suppl 4):269–279.
17 Leiblum SR (ed): Principles and practice of sex therapy, ed 4. New York, The Guilford Press, 2007.
18 Basson R: Sexuality in chronic illness. Lancet 2007;369:350–352.
19 Basson R, Schultz WW: Sexual sequelae of general medical disorders. Lancet 2007;369:409–424.
20 Levine SB (ed): Handbook of clinical sexuality for mental health professionals. New York, Brunner-Routledge, Taylor & Francis Books, 2003.
21 Balon R, Segraves RT: Handbook of sexual dysfunction. Boca Raton, Florida, Taylor & Francis, 2005.
22 Bancroft J, Loftus J, Long JS: Distress about sex: a national survey of women in heterosexual relationships. Arch Sex Behav 2003;32:193–208.
23 Balon R, Segraves RT, Clayton A: Issues for DSM-V: sexual dysfunction, disorder, or variation along normal distribution: toward rethinking DSM criteria of sexual dysfunctions. Am J Psychiatry 2007;164: 198–200.
24 Balon R: The DSM criteria of sexual dysfunction: need for a change. J Sex Marital Ther 2008; in press.
25 Prause N, Graham CA: Asexuality: classification and characterization. Arch Sex Behav 2007;36:341–356.
26 DeRogatis LR, Burnett LR: Key methodological issues in sexual medicine research. J Sex Med 2007; 4:527–537.

Richard Balon, MD
UPC-Jefferson, 2751 E. Jefferson #200
Detroit, MI 48207 (USA)
Tel. +1 313 993 3416, Fax +1 313 993 3421, E-Mail rbalon@wayne.edu

Balon R (ed): Sexual Dysfunction. The Brain-Body Connection.
Adv Psychosom Med. Basel, Karger, 2008, vol 29, pp 7–22

Clinical and Research Evaluations of Sexual Dysfunctions

Leonard R. Derogatis

Center for Sexual Medicine at Sheppard Pratt and Department of Psychiatry,
Johns Hopkins University School of Medicine, Baltimore, Md., USA

Abstract

Evaluations of the nature of an individual's sexual functioning are done with relative frequency in today's clinical healthcare environment, often prompted by sequelae of a medical disorder (e.g. diabetes, breast cancer), surgical procedure (e.g. bilateral oophorectomy), or prescribed medications (SSRI antidepressant, antihypertensive). In addition, an increasingly large number of evaluations of sexual functioning are done in association with clinical trials research in the rapidly emerging field of sexual medicine. Although clinical and research assessments of sexual functioning share many similarities, they can also be quite different, with distinct perspectives and goals regarding the assessment process. Research evaluations tend to be narrowly focused on an index condition, with highly defined patient characteristics, and long lists of inclusion/exclusion criteria. Treatment regimens are defined by research protocol a priori, and assigned through randomization, with few options for alternatives. The process results in a rigorously defined sample of patients, but one that may be hard to generalize from to real world clinical reality. Clinical sexual evaluations, on the other hand, tend to arise in a much broader health context. There are no exclusionary patient characteristics; medical, psychological, and relationship complexities all form the context in which the patient's sexual functioning occurs, and must be factored in to the clinical evaluation and treatment recommendations. Regardless of which context gives rise to the evaluation, there are three basic sources of data that we draw from: psychometric assessment, clinical interview and laboratory assays. The clinician doing a sexual evaluation must assimilate and integrate the data from these three sources in an iterative process and arrive at a cogent diagnosis and treatment plan.

In the clinical context, an 'evaluation' typically refers to an appraisal or assessment of some domain(s) of an individual's health status. In the case of the current discourse, the domain of interest is the individual's *sexual functioning*. Evaluation may be defined as, 'a specified set of operations designed to examine and determine the state of an individual's health status, usually, with the purpose of defining a benchmark, making an assessment of morbidity (i.e. a diagnosis), or establishing a need for, or the optimal course of, a therapeutic intervention'.

Sexual dysfunction is a highly prevalent condition, with prevalence showing a definite relationship to age and health status for both men and women [1]. From the outset, however, I believe it is important to make a distinction between 'clinical' and 'research' evaluations of sexual dysfunction. This distinction is important because while there is definite overlap between the methods of assessment used in these two evaluation contexts, their perspectives, purposes and goals are often quite dissimilar.

My major reason for highlighting this distinction between research and clinical evaluations is that traditionally, often via a somewhat opaque translational process, the results derived from clinical research are regularly incorporated into, and frequently become the basis for, standard clinical practice. This being the case, I believe it is important to understand the nature and scope of the differences between research and clinical evaluative processes.

Research evaluations tend to be focused on defining the presence or absence and relative severity or status of a specified *index* condition in the patient. The condition and its treatment are usually the major focus of the research program. Typically, a comprehensive baseline screening process rules out patients with comorbid conditions, prohibitive medications, laboratory values outside the normal range, a medical history of certain conditions (e.g. cancer, psychiatric disorders) and undesired physical, relational, or demographic status (e.g. BMI greater than 35, impaired personal relationship, age greater than 70). Research evaluations, initiated at 'baseline' continue to be done systematically throughout the course of the research study, although the baseline and 'final visit' assessments are usually the most comprehensive. Evaluations for any treatment-emergent adverse events are added once treatment has been initiated. Research evaluations are typically very much bound by the context of the index condition and its treatment. Other aspects of the patient's sexual functioning, medical, and psychological status are addressed only insomuch as they may have a measurable effect on the research condition of note. The research sexual evaluation should be appreciated as a much more narrowly focused assessment, with a very highly defined sample of patients, compared to clinical sexual evaluations.

Clinical sexual evaluations on the other hand, while also focused on the nature and scope of an individual's sexual morbidity, do so within a much broader overall health context. Patients are not dismissed from the evaluation because of medical, psychological, or relational complexities, but rather these events must be taken into account and factored into the clinical evaluation and recommendations for treatment. This being the case, clinical evaluations sometimes involve assessments in greater depth than research evaluations, although the sequential follow-up evaluations built into typical research protocols are usually not part of the patient's appraisal. The principal goal of most clinical evaluations is to determine the patient's diagnosis, and an optimum treatment regimen. By contrast, the patient's diagnosis is usually specified a priori in operational research protocols, which also specify the nature and magnitude of any treatments. Although many of the same operations comprise both research and clinical evaluations, the logistic and operational features of the assessments, and their primary goals, are usually quite distinct. In research evaluations, the patient's status is specified a priori to a high degree. Diagnosis is indicated by the protocol, and the ultimate purpose of evaluation is usually to determine the efficacy and safety of a specified treatment, also established a priori, in treating patients with that diagnosis. In clinical evaluations we are usually working with patients de novo. Nothing is specified or known a priori except the presenting complaint, and at the very least, a focused review of systems within the medical history must be done as well as obtaining a comprehensive sexual history.

Regardless of whether our evaluation occurs within the clinical or research context, there are basically three fundamental sources of data from which we can draw our conclusions: psychometric assessment, clinical interview, laboratory assays. Most data in our evaluations derive from the first two sources, with occasional insights or clarification drawn from laboratory test results. In the sections that follow I will try to outline in some depth each of these three principal evaluative resources and advance a paradigm for articulating the data developed from each source.

Psychometric Assessment

One of the three primary sources of potential information about a patient's sexual functioning is psychometric assessment. Psychometric assessment may take the form of self-report inventories, clinical rating scales, or structured interviews. Regardless of the particular measurement modality utilized, all assessments are designed to enable the clinician to score and quantify the patient's report, usually across multiple domains or dimensions of sexual functioning (e.g. sexual desire, arousal), and in the case of some measures, generate an overall or aggregate sexual functioning score. Although psychological measurement is sometimes misconstrued as 'soft' or 'unscientific', this disapprobation is clearly unwarranted in the case of *validated* psychological measures. The development of such measures is as much governed by the laws of science as the development of any form of physical measurement. The limitation of psychometrics has to do with its *precision* not its science, principally because it is predominantly utilized to quantify hypothetical constructs (e.g. sexual desire, depression, anxiety) instead of physical variables (e.g. weight, distance) [2]. The validation of psychological measures is accomplished by a highly prescribed set of operations and stages. It also tends to be programmatic in nature, constantly redefining and expanding, via evidence-based studies, the validation statement for the instrument [3].

The majority of measures used to accomplish psychological assessment tend to be self-report inventories, although occasional structured interviews are also employed. Self-report scales tend to be brief, inexpensive and easy to use, and may be administered by nurses, technicians or administrative personnel. Little or no specialized orientation or training is required to administer and process these measures, and many of them come with actuarial criteria to facilitate interpreting scores. In the context of clinical research trials, they are typically utilized as primary and secondary outcomes measures. In the context of clinical assessment, they find high application in primary care as screening measures for sexual dysfunction, and in more specialized contexts as an additional mechanism to help understand the nature and magnitude of patients' sexual problems.

Specific Measures of Sexual Function

In the section that follows and through summary information in table 1, I have tried to provide information on 7 validated contemporary instruments designed to assess and quantify the quality of an individual's sexual functioning. I have also included the Female Sexual Distress Scale (FSDS) which, although it is not strictly speaking a measure of sexual function/dysfunction, has become something of a standard in the field. The FSDS is a unidimensional measure of sexually-related personal distress among women, the presence of which must be established before a DSM-IV diagnosis can be assigned. All of the measures reviewed have been created relatively recently, with the majority having been developed and validated during the past decade. These instruments vary in terms of modality of measurement, breadth of assessment, and gender appropriateness; however, all have performed well against established psychometric criteria and have sound empirical evidence of reliability and validity.

The *Derogatis Interview for Sexual Functioning* (DISF/DISF-SR) is a coordinated set of brief instruments designed to provide an estimate of the quality of an individual's current sexual functioning [4]. The DISF is semi-structured interview composed of 25 items which represents quality of sexual functioning in a multidomain format. The DISF-SR is a matching self-report inventory intended to accomplish the same goal in a patient self-report mode. Gender-specific versions of the DISF and the DISF-SR exist for both males and females. All instruments in the DISF series are designed to be interpreted at three distinct levels: discrete items, functional domains, and aggregate summary score. DISF items are arranged into five primary domains of sexual functioning: sexual cognition/fantasy, sexual arousal, sexual behavior/experience, orgasm, and sexual drive/relationship. In addition, an aggregate DISF total score is computed which summarizes quality of sexual functioning across the five primary DISF domains. Both the DISF and the DISF-SR take approximately 12–15 min to administer, with the interview usually taking a few minutes longer. Internal consistency reliabilities for measures of the DISF-SR are well within acceptable ranges, as are test-retest temporal stability coefficients. Interrater reliability estimates for the DISF interview were also very good. The DISF/DISF-SR has shown good discriminative validity and sensitivity to treatment-induced changes in both male and female versions, and gender-keyed norms (in terms of area T scores) are available for all versions of the measure. The DISF/DISF-SR are currently available in 12 languages.

The *Female Sexual Functioning Index* (FSFI)© is a brief, (19-item) self-report inventory designed to measure the quality of female sexual functioning. The FSFI represents sexual functioning on five primary dimensions of sexuality plus an aggregate total score. The FSFI was initially validated on a clinically diagnosed sample of women with female sexual arousal disorder. Subsequently, the validation statement was extended to include women with a primary clinical diagnosis of inhibited female orgasm disorder or hypoactive sexual desire disorder (HSDD) [5]. Internal consistency reliability coefficients were reported to be high (all ≥0.90) in the former study and in the acceptable range in the latter. Discriminant validity (i.e. patients versus controls) of the FSFI was clearly demonstrated in both studies, as was confirmation of divergent validity.

The *Index of Premature Ejaculation* (IPE) is a contemporary self-report inventory that focuses on the subjective aspects of the premature ejaculation experience, serving as a complement to the elapsed time measures which form the basis of intravaginal ejaculatory latency time (IELT). The IPE was created via a number of major stages, involving developing the item pool for the prototype, content analysis through patient interviews, and sequential quantitative psychometric analyses. The process resulted in reducing the 17-item prototype to a final 10-item version [6]. As part of the psychometric analysis, the IPE was subjected to factor analysis based upon a sample of 85 men. Initially, four factors, accounting for approximately 59% of the variance were observed; however, after subsequent evaluation, only three were retained: sexual satisfaction, control, and distress. A slightly modified principal component analysis was done on the 10-item version, and a three-factor solution was observed. The IPE has been shown to possess very good discriminant validity (known groups) and good convergent validity, correlating well with IELT. The IPE also showed high reliabilities, with internal consistency (coefficients alpha) ranging from 0.70 to 0.86 for the three domain scores and test-retest reliabilities varying between 0.72 and 0.83.

The *International Index of Erectile Function* (IIEF) is a 15-item self-report inventory developed by Rosen et al. [7] to make available a brief measure of erectile function and capacity. It has been frequently recommended as a primary endpoint in clinical trials of erectile dysfunction (ED), and has become a standard in that regard. The IIEF was developed in conjunction with the clinical trial program for sildenafil (Viagra), and has since served as a major endpoint in over 50 clinical trials [7]. At present, it has been linguistically validated in over 32 languages. The IIEF represents quality of male sexual function in terms of 5 domain scores: erectile function, orgasmic function, sexual desire, sexual satisfaction, and overall satisfaction. It does not possess a total score. Both internal consistency and test-retest reliabilities are superior for the IIEF, and the principal domains have been confirmed through factor analysis. Sensitivity and specificity are also very good, and concurrent validation

Table 1. Descriptive and psychometric properties of 8 contemporary measures of quality of sexual function

Inventory name	Modality/ gender	Items	Admin. time min	Domains
DISF-SR	CI and SR/male and female	25	<15	cognition, arousal, behavior, orgasm, drive/ relationship total score
FSFI	SR/female only	19	15	desire, arousal, lubrication, orgasm, satisfaction, pain
IPE	SR/male only	10	<10	sexual satisfaction, control, distress
IIEF	SR/male only	15	<15	erectile function, orgasm, desire, intercourse satisfaction, overall
PFSF	SR/female only	37	<20	desire, arousal, orgasm, pleasure, concerns, responsivenes, self-image
SFQ	SR/female only	26	<15	desire, arousal-sensation, arousal-lubrication, enjoyment, orgasm, dyspareunia, partner, total
SIDI	CI	13	<15	overall total score
FSDS/FSDS-R	SR/female only	12/13	<5	unidimensional scale measuring sexually-related personal distress; R version has an additional desire item

SR = Self-report; CI = clinical interview.

against other comparable measures has been shown. Discriminative validity has been well established in comparisons of functional versus dysfunctional samples, and sensitivity to therapeutic change has been robustly demonstrated within the context of clinical trials of sildenafil and other treatments for ED. More recently, a 5-item brief form of the IIEF termed the Sexual Health Inventory for Men has been developed and validated [8].

In the developmental strategy for the *Profile of Female Sexual Functioning* (PFSF) [9, 10], preliminary items and domains of sexual function were identified through interviews with surgically and naturally menopausal women in both the United States and Europe. A subset of items was selected for translation and further analysis. The resulting instrument is a self-report inventory developed by Procter & Gamble Pharmaceuticals to serve as a major outcomes measure in their trials of Intrinsa, a new transdermal testosterone treatment system for women suffering from low sexual desire. Qualitative linguistic validation was conducted in women with HSDD and non-HSDD women in eight countries to ensure items would have the same meaning across languages. The resulting instrument was evaluated in 332 oophorectomized women with HSDD and 258 age-matched nonoophorectomized controls. Psychometric item analyses resulted in 37 items organized into seven domains (sexual desire,

Reliability			Discriminative validity		Sens./spec.	Published norms
IC (α)	TRT (r)	IRR	funct/dys.	therap. chg.		
0.74–080	0.80–0.90	0.84–0.92	yes	yes	0.89/0.7	yes
0.82	0.79–0.86	–	yes	yes	–	yes
0.74–0.91	0.70–0.90		yes	yes	–	no
0.73–0.95	0.64–0.84	–	yes	yes	0.97/0.88	yes
0.87–0.96	0.62–0.84	–	yes	yes	0.86/0.93	no
0.79–0.91	0.42–0.78	–	yes	yes	–	yes
0.90	–	–	yes	yes	–	no
0.93	0.87–0.93	–	yes	yes	0.93/0.93	yes cut-off score(s)

arousal, orgasm, sexual pleasure, sexual concerns, sexual responsiveness, and sexual self-image), which thoroughly described female sexual function in menopausal women with HSDD. Excellent reliability and validity of the domains of the PFSF were observed in all countries evaluated. Statistically significant differences between oophorectomized women with low libido and control women were found for all domains and all geographies, providing strong evidence of discriminative validity for the PFSF. In addition, measures of test-retest and internal consistency reliability were well within accepted limits. The PFSF is an instrument specifically designed for measurement of sexual desire in women with low libido. Robust psychometric properties have been established in numerous geographies and languages, making it useful for assessing therapeutic change in multinational clinical trials. A brief form of the PFSF has also recently been developed [11]. Historically, the PFSF has been treated as a proprietary instrument by Procter and Gamble Pharmaceuticals; however, the company has very recently made it available to individuals in the health care professions.

The *Sexual Function Questionnaire* (SFQ) is a self-report inventory designed as an outcomes measure of female sexual function [12]. It is composed of 26 items reflecting all aspects of the sexual response cycle – desire, arousal and orgasm – as well as dyspareunia. The item content was generated from the collective responses of 82 women to a semi-structured interview. Factor analysis yielded seven domains of female sexual function: desire, physical arousal-sensation, physical arousal-lubrication, enjoyment, orgasm, dyspareunia and partner relationship. The item content of the SFQ was reviewed by an external panel of clinicians with expertise in psychology, physiology, gynecology, physical medicine, and the treatment of FSD. Internal consistency of the domains ranged from 0.79 to 0.91 for all domains except partner relationship, which was 0.65, and test-retest reliability is in the acceptable range.

Validation studies to date include (1) two 12-week randomized, controlled clinical trials evaluating sildenafil citrate treatment vs. placebo in pre- and postmenopausal women with a diagnosis of FSD that included FSAD (n = 781), and (2) two normative 4-week trials in age-matched pre- and postmenopausal women without symptoms of FSD (n = 201). Women in these studies were aged 18–69 years.

Discriminant validity was demonstrated with a significant difference between baseline mean SFQ domain scores of women with FSD compared to women without FSD ($p < 0.0001$). Sensitivity to therapeutically induced change over time was established via evaluation of a global efficacy question in both clinical studies. Substantial significant difference was evident between positive and negative responders to this question.

The *Sexual Interest and Desire Inventory* (SIDI) is a brief, clinician-administered rating scale focused on measuring severity and change in response to treatment of HSDD in premenopausal women. The SIDI was developed in part through IRT analysis, with an initial prototype of 17-items [13], which has since been paired down to a 13-item rating scale [14]. Reports have shown the SIDI to have high internal consistency reliability (coefficient alpha = 0.90), with demonstrated discriminant validity (known groups) relative to cases versus noncases of HSDD. It has also shown good convergent validity with domains from the FSFI in the same study sample. The SIDI boasts a unique measurement format in that items address both intensity and frequency of sexual events.

The *Female Sexual Distress Scale* (FSDS) was developed to quantify and measure the construct of sexually related personal distress [15]. The presence of manifest distress in presenting patients has been a required criterion for a diagnosis of FSD in the DSM-IV system; however, no operational mechanism for quantifying distress has been previously described. Additionally, in the FDA's most recent guidance on clinical drug trials in FSD [16], the agency has made documentation of manifest personal distress a requirement for patient inclusion in clinical treatment trials.

The FSDS is a 12-item unidimensional self-report inventory designed to measure the construct of sexually-related personal distress. Repeated factor analyses of clinical trial samples have established the factorial invariance of the 12-item representation of the test, and the fact that it is unidimensional in nature. Discriminant validity studies have been done with two samples of women with HSDD, one surgical, the other natural, versus women with no sexual complaint. In the natural menopause group, a cut score of ≥15 resulted in sensitivity = 0.81, specificity = 0.93 and PVP = 0.91; in the surgical menopausal group: sensitivity = 0.93, specificity = 0.93, and PVP = 0.89 using the same cut score.

Comprehensive reliability analyses have been accomplished on the FSDS in several phase III study samples. In one clinical drug trial (n = 190), the internal consistency coefficient (alpha) was 0.93, while the test-retest correlation was 0.83 over a 4-week period. In a separate nondrug study (n = 145) involving surgically and naturally menopausal women with FSD, internal consistency coefficients ranged from 0.93 to 0.94, while test-retest (4 weeks) ranged from 0.82 to 0.84 [15].

Sensitivity to therapeutically induced change was also dramatically demonstrated in a separate trial of an agent to treat female sexual arousal disorder. Comparisons of baseline scores on the FSDS compared to those at final visit revealed very dramatic reductions in personal distress across the study period ($p < 0.001$).

The FSDS is a very brief (approximately 5 min), psychometrically sound instrument that is very easy to use. It has shown excellent ability to discriminate between FSD patients and nonpatients, as well as sensitivity to therapeutically induced change. It has been used in HSDD samples and women suffering from FSAD, with numerous different pharmacologic agents.

It is important to recognize that in spite of the fact that diagnostic-like domain labels and dimension names may suggest that diagnosis can be accomplished via psychometric instruments, particularly in the case of self-report scales, this is not the case. Psychometric assessment of the kind described here is designed to provide a quantitative snapshot of the individual's quality of sexual functioning. In most instances, it will enable us to appreciate an outline of the person's sexual function profile, and/or whether or not the individual manifests symptoms at a level consistent with a diagnosable condition. In research assessments, it represents a quantification along a dimension of functioning that, although it is clearly related to diagnosis, is not synonymous with it. Formal diagnosis of sexual dysfunction requires, in addition to presenting complaint, both historical and contemporary perspectives on such important factors as medical history, drug history, psychological and affective status, quality of relationship(s) and psychiatric history. These comprehensive data cannot be easily determined except through thorough clinical interview.

Nonetheless, psychometric assessment is essential to clinical trials outcomes research, and can also be very useful to the busy clinician attempting to identify sexual dysfunction in his/her practice. In this review, I have tried to provide a sampling of the psychometric instruments currently available to measure and quantify the status of an individual's sexual functioning. Psychometrics has progressed dramatically in sexual medicine during the past decade to a field of measurement in which a great deal of new development has taken place. Much of the impetus for the growth of measurement in this field has been provided by the pharmaceutical industry as part of their efforts to develop validated outcomes measures for the clinical trials of their new therapeutic agents. Even so, psychometric evaluation represents a potentially valid and useful source of information about an individual's sexual functioning in any evaluative context, particularly in light of the very small expense and brief effort required to conduct these assessments.

Clinical Interview

Clinical interview is the second major source of information available to us in doing clinical evaluations of sexual functioning. The clinical interview is extremely important in both research and clinical contexts; however, interviews are conducted in a somewhat different manner in research trials versus clinical practice.

Clinical Research Interview

In research trials, the 'interview' is actually almost always a series of interviews usually done by different members of the research team to establish and verify the patients' status and whether or not they qualify for the study being conducted. An initial screening interview, typically done by phone, frequently serves as a gross filter to establish certain patient characteristics. Age, gender, education, marital status, length of relationship, inclusion criteria, the absence of exclusionary characteristics, and whether or not the patient meets other study requisites are usually reviewed during the screening interview. Subsequent in-person interviews verify the data determined from the screening interview, and in addition, establish certain patient physical parameters, such as height, weight, BMI, blood pressure, medical history, drug history, and current health status. Usually, a sexual medicine expert then does a diagnostic interview to establish and verify that the patient is suffering from the index condition, and is free of any comorbid manifestations that might disqualify him/her from the study. Laboratory specimens are also collected at this time to be evaluated as further evidence of inclusion/exclusion qualifications for the patient. Essentially, the research interview is conducted with the purpose of establishing that the patient is suffering from the condition which represents the index diagnosis in the study, meets all other study criteria, and is free of any history or current condition that would prohibit him/her from study participation.

Clinical Practice Interview

As alluded to earlier, in clinical practice the patient presents without any previous screening information, unless he or she is a regular patient of the health care provider, who has previous knowledge of the condition in question. In clinical practice, for all intents and purposes, the clinical evaluation never *disqualifies* the patient from participating in treatment, unless in completing the evaluation the provider discovers a more serious condition (e.g. acute hypertension, gynecological cancer) that takes precedence over the sexual problem, and requires a more immediate intervention. Basically, the evaluation is designed to provide an ever-widening circle of accumulating evidence on health-related factors that, either in consort or independently, may be viable etiologic factors regarding the patient's current condition.

It is at least worth mentioning here that not all sexual problems meet the criteria for sexual *dysfunctions*; sometimes patients experience sexual tribulations that do not qualify for formal diagnosis, but are better characterized as sexual *difficulties*. As examples, disagreements among partners concerning how often to have intercourse (given a reasonable normative range), or when during the day to have sex, or what positions or sexual activities to try, do not truly qualify as *dysfunctions*, but are much more productively treated as *difficulties*. They reflect inclinations concerning sexual activities that are not rooted in pathophysiology or psychopathology, but rather in differing personal preferences. There is little value in invoking a medical model to try to address such issues, since usually they can be resolved through negotiation between the partners involved. Occasionally, a provider can provide useful information or education in such instances, but the concept of *treatment* is not appropriate.

Returning to the sphere of true clinical disorders, it is important to remember that etiologic factors arising from numerous biological, psychological, interpersonal and cultural origins can be operational in cases of sexual dysfunction. It is also appears that these agents do not operate independently or in a mutually exclusive manner. Rather, various etiological mechanisms tend to operate co inductively, so that multi ple factors usually contribute to any particular case of sexual dysfunction. A female sexual pain disorder, with its basis in menopause-induced changes, can give rise to a perception of 'withholding' on the part of the male partner, which if communicated, can induce anger and guilt in the female patient associated with the idea that she has failed to be 'a good lover'. ED, with origins in vascular endothelial lesions will often present with a secondary (ego-protective) manifestation of sexual disinterest, which can be interpreted by the female partner as evidence of a loss of affection and interest in her as a sexual partner. The important concern to be exercised here is that even if one can accurately identify a primary etiologic agent in a particular case, it does not eliminate the possibility of corollary factors that need to be addressed.

In figure 1, I have taken the liberty of condensing the myriad of potential sources that can have an etiological bearing on sexual functioning into three broad classes: biological, psychological, and interpersonal. In doing so, I am aware that influences from other spheres beyond these three can act causally relative to sexual dysfunction; however, I believe the majority of causal agents are subsumed under these three broad categories, and that more esoteric influences account for only a small proportion of the prevalence of sexual dysfunctions.

The first broad category outlined in figure 1 is biological. There exist an extremely large number of diseases, disorders and biological derangements that can act to produce sexual dysfunction. Causal agents range from endocrinopathies such as hyperprolactinemia, and age-related hypogonadism, through numerous chronic illnesses

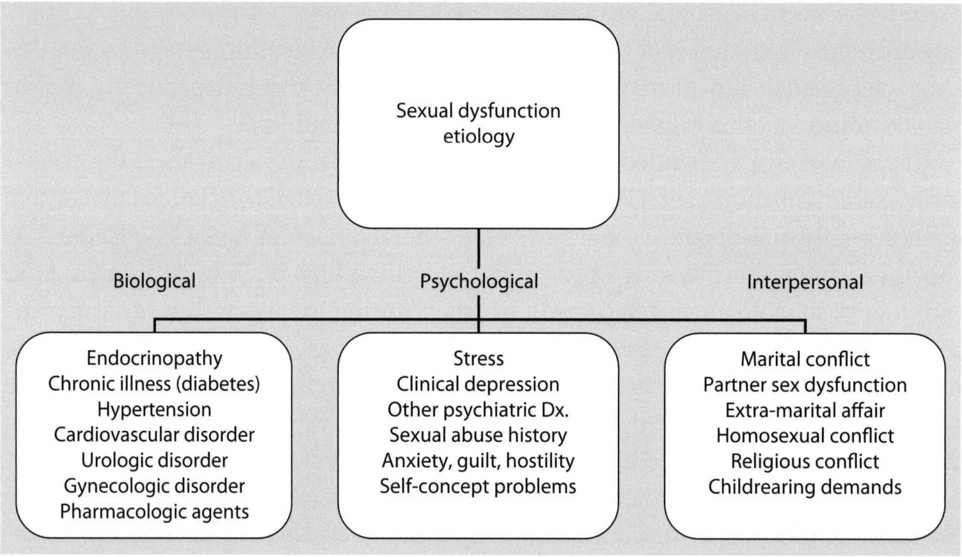

Fig. 1. Biological, psychological and interpersonal factors etiologic in sexual dysfunction.

like diabetes and cardiovascular disorders, to medical conditions that directly affect the genital organs. In addition, a vast array of pharmacologic agents, with SSRI antidepressants and antihypertensives heading the list, possess the capacity to inhibit normal sexual functioning at every stage of the sexual response cycle. As an example of the potential magnitude of medication-induced dysfunction, it is well established that the SSRI antidepressants have a prevalence of sexual dysfunction associated with them of 35–65% [17]. This is why it is extremely important, whenever possible, to conduct a thorough physical examination and review of systems, and take a careful history of medication use with particular attention to the temporal relationship between medication initiation and the onset of sexual symptoms. When they are present, biological etiologies tend to be primary in nature because they assault and undermine the fundamental biological matrix essential for the adequate performance of sexual behaviors. As I have emphasized, however, they are often not the sole etiological agent acting in a particular case.

The second class of etiological precursors identified tend to be classified as *psychological* in nature. The ubiquitous experience of stress, if it is of sufficient magnitude or duration, clinical depression, and other psychiatric disorders, are all associated with the presence of sexual dysfunction, with clinical depression having an established prevalence rate of 40–50% [18]. An individual does not have to be afflicted with a formal psychiatric disorder, however, for psychological factors to play a disruptive role in his/her sexual function. Any strong negative affect state, e.g. anxiety, guilt, hostility can be extremely disruptive to effective and satisfying sexual function. Sex works best in a relaxed state of mind, and negative emotions have the effect of distracting the individual from appropriate sexual cognitions, and disrupting the smooth progression of sexual arousal from early initial levels through high plateau and eventual orgasm. Often, such negative emotions are associated with chronic self-concept problems, where the individual has heightened concern about some aspect of his or her physical or psychological person. Such conflicts can range widely, from concerns regarding physical adequacy and attractiveness (e.g. body image), to intrapsychic conflicts about fear of disease or pregnancy. The goal in the clinical interview is to ascertain that such conflicts exist, with the treatment of such problems often accomplished through referral to a specialist.

The final broad class of potential etiologic agents in sexual dysfunction I have labeled *interpersonal*, because, for the most part, they arise from conflicted interactions within the individual's interpersonal relationships. It goes without saying, that such conflicts usually give rise to strong negative emotions. Marital conflict represents a more or less generic label for any of the hundreds, if not thousands, of controversies that couples find themselves engaged in from time to time. Usually, it is not the substantive aspect of the argument that interferes with sexual intimacy, but rather the negative emotions that the partners harbor or direct at each other. At other times it *is* the specific conflicted issue that holds the disruptive potential. Conflicts revolving around extra-marital liaisons, or sexual disinterest arising from homosexual preferences are just two specific examples. In addition, childrearing can at times fall disproportionately to one or another parent, producing considerable dismay and resentment. Clinicians should also be sensitive to the possibility that partner sexual dysfunctions exist, which are not addressed by the patient, often out of embarrassment, or a misconstrued belief that the partner's dysfunction actually represents disinterest in them as a sexual partner.

Laboratory Assays

Although laboratory assays are occasionally definitive in determining the etiologic picture (e.g. hyperprolactinemia associated with a pituitary adenoma), for the most part they rule biologic factors in or out of the diagnostic equation. The critical question with laboratory assays often comes down to cost/benefit in the broadest sense of that concept. That is to say, what is the incremental value of adding a particular test to the laboratory request, and the probability that it will identify a significant causal agent. This increment must be weighed against the cost in time and energy required to obtain and interpret the test result, and the dollar cost associated with the assay.

Often, clinicians are discouraged from ordering any but the most basic laboratory tests because published data based on the general population show that the 'hit rate' or probability of a positive is relatively small. It is important to remember, however, that by virtue of their presenting complaint, sexually dysfunctional patients no longer

Table 2. Recommended laboratory assays useful in the diagnosis of sexual dysfunctions

Recommended diagnostic assays	Optional diagnostic assays
Plasma estradiol	Lipid profile
Total testosterone	DHEA
Free testosterone	Fasting glucose
SHBG	HbA1C
TSH	Thyroid panel
Prolactin	LH and FSH CBC

SHBG = Sex hormone-binding globulin; TSH = thyroid-stimulating hormone; DHEA = dehydroepiandrosterone; HbA1C = glycosylated hemoglobin A1C; LH = luteinizing hormone; FSH = follicle-stimulating hormone; CBC = complete blood count.

represent the 'general' population, but are now members of a specific subset of individuals where the probability (i.e. the 'base rate') of a sexually-related biological derangement is much higher. This is particularly true if the individual under evaluation is over 50 years of age.

One can find almost as many different lists of recommended laboratory tests as there are experts. Some of this variation is a result of the recommending expert's particular specialty, and the nature of the patients seen in his/her practice. Also, the patient's gender obviously plays a role in the specific labs requested, as does the patient's presenting complaint, its duration (lifelong vs. acquired) and its specificity (situational vs. generalized). In some cases, there is little to be gained from laboratory assays, for example when a woman experiences low sexual desire with her husband, but no problems with her lover. Such manifestly interpersonal etiologies tend to be rare, however, and often difficult to ascertain.

The list outlined in table 2 is a relatively generic inventory of laboratory assays that can be utilized in both male and female patients to determine if any 'first line' (relative to sexual functioning) biological functions appear abnormal. I have divided tests into 'recommended' and 'optional', very much based on what we do in our Center. It is obvious that many more assays could be added, a few subtracted, and others shifted from the 'recommended' to the 'optional' list and vice versa. Usually, laboratory tests do not provide a definitive etiology for a disorder, rather they more often give us a signal of where to look further.

Assimilation and Integration of the Data

The clinical evaluation process essentially represents an iterative progression with ever-increasing quantities of data concerning the patient's presenting complaint, sexual, medical and interpersonal histories, and summary of current assessments. The clinician's principal task is to assimilate these data and integrate the multiple elements into a cohesive assessment and explanation of the nature of the patient's sexual dysfunction and its probable cause(s). There are a number of important issues that should be kept in mind during this process.

First, the evaluation should be perceived by the clinician, and explained to the patient, as being a programmatic endeavor; it is not a one-shot, all or none process, but rather a complementary series of assessments that will hopefully result in a comprehensive understanding of the patient's problem, and an optimum approach to treatment. This being the case, whenever possible the patient's partner should be involved in the evaluation so that he/she can provide verification and corroboration of the facts of the case, and at the time of treatment recommendations or referral also help confirm the whys and wherefores of the clinician's recommendations.

Second, in the current era of patient-based medicine it is important that the patient (and the patient's partner whenever possible) be perceived and treated as important decision makers in the evaluation and treatment process. The clinician should be careful not to assume an authoritarian posture, but rather take on the role of an expert guide, informing, educating, and sharing knowledge and experience with the patient, and ultimately sharing details concerning accepting a referral or initiating a particular treatment regimen. Since education represents a critical aspect of the evaluation process, the patient should be exposed to the data comprising the various clinical assessments, and the processes whereby these data impact on the clinician's decision making and recommendations regarding the case.

Data from the patient's psychometric assessment, clinical interview and laboratory assays should be shared with the patient in an effort to have him/her understand the basis for the conclusions that the clinician has reached. These data and their assimilation by the provider will form the platform for the clinician's treatment recommendations. Since the patient should be an active participant in decisions to accept or reject specific treatment recommendations, it is essential that the patient understand the nature of the data the clinician has used in his decision-making.

In many cases, it is possible that the primary care provider can initiate and maintain effective treatment for the patient's sexual dysfunction, but this is not always the case. Underlying complex cardiovascular or endocrine conditions, male or female disorders requiring surgery for optimal resolution, and psychiatric or interpersonal conflicts that demand specialized treatment knowledge, all represent situations where a referral should be made. If referral turns out to be the case, it is important that the primary care provider maintain communication both with the patient about how treatment has progressed, and the specialist to promote an integrated treatment program.

Optimal treatment is the ultimate goal of the clinical evaluation process, whether it is delivered by the primary care clinician or a specialized health care provider. The more relevant information that can be brought to bear in the evaluation process, the greater likelihood that the most appropriate treatment of the problem will be achieved.

References

1 Derogatis LR, Burnett AL: The epidemiology of sexual dysfunctions. J Sex Med 2008;5:289–300.

2 Nunnally JC: Psychometric theory. New York, NY, McGraw-Hill, 1978.

3 Derogatis LR: Assessment of sexual function/dysfunction via patient reported outcomes. Int J Impot Res 2008; in press.

4 Derogatis LR: The Derogatis Interview for Sexual Functioning (DISF/DISF-SR):An introductory report. J Sex Marital Ther 1997;23:291–304.

5 Rosen R, Brown C, Heiman J, Leiblum S, Meston C, Shabsigh R, Ferguson D, D'Agostino D: The Female Sexual Function Index (FSFI): A multidimensional self-report instrument for the assessment of female sexual function. J Sex Mar Ther 2000;26:191–208.

6 Althof S, Rosen R, Symonds T, Mundayat R, May K, Abraham L: Development and validation of a new questionnaire to assess sexual satisfaction, control and distress associated with premature ejaculation. J Sex Med 2006;3:465–475.

7 Rosen R, Riley A, Wagner G, Osterloh IH, Kirkpatrick J, Mishra A: The International Index of Erectile Function (IIEF): A multidimensional scale for assessment of sexual dysfunction. Urology 1997;49: 822–830.

8 Rosen R, Cappelleri JC, Gendrano N: The International Index of Erectile Function (IIEF): A state of the science review. Int J Impot Res 2002;14:226–244.

9 Derogatis LR, Rust J, Golombok S, Davis S, Bouchard N, Rodenberg C: Validation of the Profile of Female Sexual Function (PFSF) in surgically and naturally menopausal women. J Sex Marital Ther 2004; 30:25–36.

10 McHorney CA, Rust J, Golombok S, Davis S, Bouchard C, Rodenberg C, Derogatis LR: Profiles of female sexual function: a patient-based, international psychometric instrument for the assessment of hypoactive sexual desire in oophorectomized women. Menopause 2004;11:1–10.

11 Rust J, Derogatis LR, Rodenberg C, Koochaki P, Schmidt S, Golombok S: Development and validation of a new screening tool for hypoactive sexual desire disorder: The Brief Profile of Female Sexual Function (B-PFSF). Gynecol Endocrinol 2007;23:638–644.

12 Quirk FH, Heiman J, Rosen RC, Laan E, Smith MD, Boolel M: Development of a sexual function questionnaire for clinical trials of female sexual function. J Womens Health Gend Based Med 2002;11:277–285.

13 Sills T, Wunderlich G, Ryke R, Segraves RT, Leiblum S, Clayton A, Cotton D, Evans K: The Sexual Interest and Desire Inventory-Female (SIDI-F): Item response analysis of data from women diagnosed with hypoactive sexual desire disorder. J Sex Med 2005;2:801–818.

14 Clayton AH, Segraves RT, Leiblum S, Basson R, Pyke R, Cotton D, Lewis-D'agostino D, Evans KR, Sills TL, Wunderlich G: Reliability and validity of the Sexual Interest and Desire Inventory-Female (SIDI-F), a scale designed to measure severity of female hypoactive sexual desire disorder. J Sex Marital Ther 2006;32:115–135.

15 Derogatis LR, Rosen RC, Leiblum S, Burnett A, Heiman J: The Female Sexual Distress Scale (FSDS): Initial validation of a standardized scale for the assessment of sexually related personal distress in women. J Sex Marital Ther 2002;28:317–330.

16 U.S. Department of Health and Human Services, Food and Drug Administration, Center for Drug Evaluation and Research (CDER), Guidance for Industry: Female Sexual Dysfunction: Clinical Development of Drug Products for Treatment. Rockville, MD, 2000.

17 Clayton A, Pradko JF, Croft HA, Montano B, Leadbetter RA, Bolden-Watson C, Bass KI, Rafe BA, Donahue MJ, Jamerson BD, Metz A: Prevalence of sexual dysfunction among newer antidepressants. J Clin Psychiatry 2002;63:357–366.

18 Bonierbale M, Lancon C, Tignol J, The ELIXIR study: Evaluation of sexual dysfunction in 4557 depressed patients in France. Curr Med Res Opin 2003;19:114–124.

Leonard R. Derogatis, PhD
Center for Sexual Medicine at Sheppard Pratt
6501 N. Charles Street
Baltimore, MD 21285-6815 (USA)
Tel. +1 410 938 4336, Fax +1 410 938 4340, E-Mail Lderogatis@sheppardpratt.org

Balon R (ed): Sexual Dysfunction. The Brain-Body Connection.
Adv Psychosom Med. Basel, Karger, 2008, vol 29, pp 23–32

Management of Hypoactive Sexual Desire Disorder

Robert Taylor Segraves

Case School of Medicine, Cleveland, Ohio, USA

Abstract

Epidemiological studies have found that problems with sexual desire are one of the most common sexual complaints in females. Such complaints are far less common in males. In women, problems with sexual desire have been found to be associated with age, relationship duration, relationship distress, and complaints of anxiety and depression. Evidence-based interventions include cognitive behavioral therapy and androgen therapy. Endocrinopathies are common causes of male problems with libido. There is minimal evidence available concerning the treatment of psychological etiologies of low sexual desire in men.

Management of Hypoactive Sexual Desire Disorder

Disorders of sexual desire are frequently encountered in psychiatric practice. These disorders may be part of the presentation of common psychiatric disorders such as depression and anxiety disorders, a drug side effect, secondary to relationship discord or idiopathic. Understanding the etiology of problems of low sexual desire is also complicated because of the interplay of biological, psychological and interpersonal influences. Because these disorders can have a multitude of etiologies, diagnosis is often complicated and most often imprecise. Because sexuality is such an important part of one's self-identity and plays a significant role in intimate relationships, low sexual desire can have a multitude of unfortunate consequences and obviously should be a focus of psychiatric interventions [1].

The goal of this chapter is to review current evidence concerning the diagnosis, epidemiology, etiology and treatment of hypoactive sexual desire disorders. Masters and Johnson [2] and the DSM-IV-TR [3] regard male and female sexual disorders as symmetrical. However, there appear to be sex differences in the strength of sexual desire, its covariates, its sequencing in the sexual response cycle, and its response to relationship discord [4]. In this chapter, female disorders of desire will be considered separately from male disorders of desire as they may represent different diagnostic entities.

Female Hypoactive Sexual Desire Disorder

Diagnosis

Modern nomenclature for the sexual disorders can be traced to Masters and Johnson [2] who delineated premature ejaculation, ejaculatory incompetence, impotence, orgasmic dysfunction, vaginismus and dyspareunia. Except for vaginismus and dyspareunia, the sexual dysfunctions were linked to the phases of the sexual response cycle (excitement, plateau, orgasm). The sexual response cycle and those disorders of sexual response were considered to be analogous in both sexes. This diagnostic scheme was initially adopted by most mental health clinicians. As more clinicians gained experience in the treatment of sexual disorders, it became increasingly obvious that the major problem of many patients was the absence of desire for sexual activity, a concept not included in the Masters and Johnson diagnostic schema. Harold Lief and Helen Singer Kaplan, both psychoanalysts, introduced this concept of the diagnosis of inhibited sexual desire [5]. The first official nomenclature for the sexual disorders was published in the DSM in 1980. In this system, inhibited sexual desire was defined as persistent and pervasive inhibition of sexual desire. The text also indicated that the diagnosis would rarely be made unless the lack of desire was a source of distress to either the individual or partner. In DSM-III-R the term inhibited was deleted as this was felt to imply a psychodynamic etiology and the somewhat awkward term, hypoactive sexual desire was substituted for inhibited sexual desire. The definition was also slightly modified. The new definition was persistently, or recurrently deficient or absent sexual fantasies and desire for sexual activity. In this edition, the following subtype modifiers were introduced: psychogenic only or psychogenic and biogenic, lifelong or acquired, generalized or situational. In DSM-IV, the definition of hypoactive sexual desire remained unchanged except for a new provision that the diagnosis could not be made unless the disturbance caused marked distress or interpersonal difficulty. This definition remained unchanged in DSM-IV-TR.

Numerous individuals and groups have criticized the DSM-IV-TR criteria for sexual disorders. Major suggestions for revision have been made by an international consensus group funded by the American Urological Association. This group met on four occasions and has published a number of manuscripts detailing recommended changes [6]. This group specifically suggested that the criteria sets for hypoactive sexual desire disorder be modified. Data indicating that many sexually responsive women do not report sexual fantasies was cited as well as evidence that some sexually responsive women do not experience desire for sexual activity but respond to sexual stimuli once involved in a sexual situation. It was recommended that lack of responsive desire be substituted for absence of desire for sexual activity. This group also noted evidence that interest in sexual activity appears to lessen both with age and relationship duration for many women. Basson [7] specifically states that the linear sequencing of desire, arousal, orgasm as outlined in DSM-IV-TR is a model better suited to male than female sexuality. She posits that many women are unaware of desire for sexual activity at the onset of sexual activity and that emotional intimacy may be the most important factor influencing a woman's initial sexual responsiveness. In this model, responsive desire and sexual arousal clearly overlap.

It should be noted that the DSM-IV-TR criteria and suggested revisions lack precise criteria sets designating severity or duration criteria. Also, the separation of sexual dysfunctions from relationship discord and adjustment disorders is imprecise. Many clinicians would not diagnose a sexual problem as a sexual dysfunction if it is clearly secondary to relationship discord. However, this is not clearly specified in the DSM-IV-TR text. Similarly, the distinction between an adjustment disorder influencing sexual function and a sexual dysfunction is not clearly specified. Precise operational criteria are necessary to define homogenous clinical groups for research and advancement of knowledge in the field.

Epidemiology

There have been numerous well-conducted epidemiological studies of the prevalence of sexual problems in the United States, Europe, and globally [8]. These studies have used differing criteria for identifying sexual problems, yet have produced somewhat similar results. Most studies have found that complaints of low desire are the most common female sexual complaint. Studies have also found that complaints of low sexual desire increase with age, relationship duration, number of small children, relationship discord and symptoms of anxiety and depression [9–11]. These studies have been criticized as not distinguishing between sexual problems (transient issues not requiring medical intervention) and sexual dysfunction (persistent, pervasive problems in adaptation requiring medical intervention).

The limitations of epidemiological data in providing estimates of the frequency of sexual dysfunction in the general population can be appreciated by a careful analysis of the most comprehensive studies to date, the Global Study of Sexual Attitudes and Behavior [8]. This study collected data from 27,500 men and women in 29 countries. Sampling techniques had to be modified for some countries such that comparisons of rates across countries is somewhat problematic. The question pertaining to low sexual desire was 'During the last 12 months have you ever experienced for a period of two months or more when you lacked interest in having sex?' If the answer was affirmative, the subject was then asked to rate its frequency as occasionally, sometimes or frequently. This study has been quoted as finding that approximately 33% of women in Canada and the United States complained of low sexual desire. However, this number represents an aggregate of all women reporting occasional, periodic and frequent problems with low libido. The number of women reporting frequent problems with libido was only 7.9%. A stratified population sample survey in the UK [12] found that approximately 41% of British females complained of lack of interest in sex for at least 1 month the previous year. However, only 10% had this problem for as long as 6 months. The DSM-IV-TR requires that the problem causes marked distress or interpersonal difficulty in order to be diagnosed as a sexual dysfunction. Very few studies have measured personal distress. The few that have monitored personal distress find that only 50% of women with sexual problems reported associated distress.

In conclusion, we have data concerning the prevalence of sexual problems in the general population. However, the prevalence of frequent, distressing problems of lack of interest in sex lasting for at least 6 months' duration is unknown.

Psychological Treatment of Hypoactive Sexual Desire Disorder

A variety of different procedures have been incorporated into what is known as cognitive behavioral therapy of low sexual desire. A mainstay of this approach is a focus on modifying dysfunctional attitudes and thoughts about sexual behavior. Another technique involves identifying distractions during sexual stimulation and then removing these distractions. The woman is asked to focus on the types of stimulation she finds pleasurable and to communicate this to her partner. Frequently, issues of fostering trust and respect in a relationship as well as restoring emotional intimacy are a necessary part of treatment. Sensate focus exercises that involve a graded transition from nonsexual to sexual touching may be employed. There is some evidence to support the efficacy of cognitive behavioral treatment for hypoactive sexual desire disorder in women [13].

Endocrinological Treatment

Interest in the use of androgens to increase libido in women dates back at least to the 1940s when clinicians observed that androgen therapy of menstrual problems resulted in increased libido [14]. In fact, a double-blind placebo-controlled study in 1950 demonstrated that whereas diethylstilbestrol decreased hot flashes, methyltestosterone increased libido [15]. In 1985, Sherwin et al. [16] reported a prospective double-blind study of the administration of testosterone in women who were after oophorectomy. In the group receiving androgen alone or androgen in combination with estrogen, there were increased scores on measures of arousal, desire and sexual fantasies. More recently, Procter and Gamble has sponsored numerous studies of the use of a testosterone patch (Intrinsa) in women after oophorectomy complaining of low sexual desire [17]. These studies have demonstrated that testosterone therapy increases libido and sexual satisfaction. One study found that acute testosterone administration increased libido in healthy eugonadal females. It is of note that two large cross-sectional studies did not find evidence of a strong relationship between measures of endogenous androgen activity and sexual function [18]. A new drug application received a negative review by the Food and Drug Administration of the United States although the patch now has approval by the European authorities for use in postmenopausal women.

Most of the studies using testosterone involved postmenopausal women and testosterone therapy was combined with estrogen replacement. Many women are concerned about the long-term effects of estrogen on the risk of breast cancer and cardiovascular disease. Topical estrogen in the form of estrogen rings and tablets greatly reduces the extent of systemic absorption and may be preferred by some women [19].

Pharmacological Approaches

Numerous companies have investigated whether compounds that facilitate erections in men might also facilitate female sexual function. The rationale for these investigations in women is that sexual arousal in women involves peripheral vasocongestion similar to penile erection in men. Most trials of drugs that promote genital vasocongestion have proved to be unsuccessful in the treatment of female sexual dysfunction. This includes α-adrenergic blockers, alprostadil, and phophodiesterase inhibitors [5]. The failure of vasoactive drugs to increase subjective sexual responsiveness in women might have been anticipated as numerous psychophysiological studies had failed to demonstrate a consistent relationship between measures of genital arousal and subjective sexual arousal in women.

Another approach has been to test possible efficacy of compounds targeting the central nervous system. This research rests on a considerable body of evidence in laboratory animals that drugs affecting dopaminergic and serotonergic pathways influence sexual behavior. Dopaminergic drugs such as levodopa and pergolide have been reported to increase sexual activity and the effect of apomorphine in women with hypoactive sexual desire disorder has been studied with mixed results [5]. Bupropion, an antidepressant with both dopamine and norepinephrine reuptake inhibition, has been found to have moderate prosexual effects in women with hypoactive sexual desire disorder [20]. Another compound being tested for the treatment of hypoactive sexual desire disorder is flibanserin, a drug with serotonin 5-HT2 antagonism and serotonin 5-HT1a agonism [21]. Melanocortin receptor agonists are being studied and have been found to increase sexual responsiveness in both men and women [22]. A number of other compounds with different mechanisms of action are being investigated.

Several products available without prescription are available in the United States market. Most of these compounds involve mixtures of herbal products. Double-blind placebo-controlled studies on poorly specified populations have been reported for most of these products including Xzite, Avlimil, Arginmax and Zestra. Evidence concerning the efficacy of dehydroepiandrosterone is also unclear.

Differential Diagnosis

Once a diagnosis of hypoactive sexual desire is made, one begins a logical process of attempting to first identify etiologies that are treatable. A useful process is to first classify the disorder by DSM-IV-TR subtypes. For example, lifelong hypoactive sexual desire disorder is strongly suggestive of a psychogenic etiology and of lifelong dysfunctional attitudes toward sexual behavior and pleasure. In such cases, a cognitive behavioral approach focusing on attitudes and thoughts about sexual expression would usually be the first intervention. If the problem is acquired after a period of normal function, lifelong attitudes about sexual behavior are unlikely to be etiologically involved as the person functioned well in the past. If the problem is acquired, the differential now turns to whether the problem is global (in all sexual situations) or situation specific (only present under certain circumstances). For obvious reasons, situation-specific problems suggest a psychogenic etiology. Global-acquired problems present greater diagnostic issues. One first attempts to identify problems treatable by commonly accepted methodologies of proven efficacy. For example, one would want to rule out depression and anxiety disorders as etiologically involved. One would want to rule out drug side effects focusing on psychiatric and antihypertensive drugs. A careful history should establish whether the difficulty is secondary to pain. Most clinicians would also rule out thyroid disease as well as hyperprolactinemia. One would want to focus carefully on the interpersonal relationship issues. If all of the above are negative, one is then faced with an idiopathic hypoactive sexual desire disorder. In such situations, one first strives to do no harm, starting with relatively benign interventions. In the absence of seizure disorder, bupropion is generally a well-tolerated drug. Next, one could consider trials of over the counter topical stimulants such as Zestra. As a last resort, one might consider off-label use of testosterone.

Male Hypoactive Sexual Desire Disorder

In the DSM-IV-TR, the same criteria apply to the diagnosis of male and female hypoactive sexual desire disorder. There have been no publications addressing whether male criteria should be modified.

Epidemiology

Epidemiological studies have found that the prevalence of complaints of low sexual desire is lower in men than women [23, 24]. In the Global Study of Sexual Attitudes and Behavior, 17.6 % of men in Canada, the United States, Australia, New Zealand, and South Africa complained of lack of sexual interest. However, only 2.7% complained of this as a frequent problem. Lack of interest in sex was associated with older age, poor health, and depression. Similarly, in a national probability sample of sexual behavior in the United Kingdom, 17% of men complained of low sexual desire in the preceding year. However, only 1.8% complained of this problem lasting for at least 6 months.

Psychological Treatment of Male Sexual Desire Disorder

As noted in the 'Epidemiology' section, male sexual desire disorder is far less common than female sexual desire disorder and less has been written concerning the psychological treatment of such disorders in men. Most of the treatment approaches involve helping the individual develop sensory awareness and to identify erotic cues in his environment, desensitization of anxiety-evoking stimuli, cognitive restructuring and couple psychotherapy [25]. Some therapists recommend a psychotherapeutic approach concentrating on transferential relationships and internalization of past exciting and rejecting objects. To the authors knowledge, there is minimal empirical support for any of these approaches [4].

Pharmacotherapy

Pharmacological approaches mainly concern the treatment of psychiatric conditions known to be associated with low sexual desire such as depression, anxiety disorders and psychotic disorders. Depression has been well established as a cause of low sexual desire and its successful treatment can lead to the restoration of libido.

Unfortunately, some of the pharmacological interventions for depression are themselves associated with sexual dysfunction, especially anorgasmia and to a lesser extent low desire [26]. This can be minimized by the use of antidepressants such as bupropion or nefazodone that are rarely associated with sexual dysfunction. There is also some evidence that duloxetine may be associated with a lower incidence of sexual dysfunction than the selective serotonin reuptake inhibitors [27]. If an SSRI is required, there is some evidence that antidotes may preserve libido [28, 29].

It is also well known that many psychotic disorders, especially schizophrenia, may be associated with decreased libido. Again, successful treatment of the psychosis may help to restore libido but many antipsychotic drugs may have sexual side effects [30]. The available evidence suggests that prolactin-sparing antipsychotic agents may have lower incidence of sexual dysfunction. Also, use of dopamine agonists such as bromocriptine and cabergoline may help lessen the side effect burden of these agents.

One study of couples with low sexual desire found that bupropion had a prosexual effect [31]. This study has not been replicated.

Endocrinological Therapy

Endocrinological therapy mainly consists of treating endocrine disorders associated with hypoactive sexual desire disorder. These primarily include hypothyroidism, hyperprolactinemia and hypogonadism. Hypothyroidism has been found to be associated with lower sexual libido and restoration of a euthyroid state has been associated with an improvement in libido. Low sexual desire along with fatigue can be presenting symptoms of hyperprolactinemia. Hyperprolactinemia is important to detect as it may be the result of a pituitary tumor. Pituitary microadenomas may respond to bromocriptine or cabergoline therapy [32].

Much of the evidence concerning the relationship of androgen levels to libido has been derived from studies of patients who are androgen deficient as the result of disease states. In hypogonadal states, most men report a marked decrease in libido that is restored by androgen replacement therapy. In patients who have been castrated, the usual sequence is first a decrease in libido followed in several weeks by a loss in the ability to ejaculate. Similar effects have been observed in men receiving antiandrogen therapy. Laboratory studies have suggested that hypogonadism is associated with decreased nocturnal erections and decreased sexual fantasies. The relationship between androgen levels and libido within the normal range is unclear. Most evidence suggests that a minimal level of androgen, perhaps slightly above the lower limit of normal is necessary to support normal sexual function and that increases in androgen above this level have negligible effects on libido in most men. However, there is reason to believe that the threshold for the biological effects of androgen in older men might be higher than in younger men. In these cases, one might attempt to achieve slightly higher serum androgen levels than one would in younger men [33].

Current recommendations are to attempt to restore serum testosterone to mid-normal range. A variety of therapeutic approaches are possible. These include 75–100 mg testosterone enanthate or cyprioate administered weekly, one to two 5 mg testosterone patches nightly, 5–10 mg of testosterone gel applied daily, or 30 mg bioadhesive buccal testosterone tablet applied every 12 h. Follow-up care should include routine PSA, hematocrit and serum testosterone levels.

Potential side effects of testosterone replacement therapy include prostatic hypertrophy, increased erythropoiesis, worsened sleep apnea, gynecomastia, and fluid retention possibly worsening hypertension and cardiac failure.

The effect of androgen on male libido decreases with age as the result of decreased testicular function, decreased activity of the hypothalamic pituitary axis, an increase in serum hormone-binding globulin decreasing the amount of bioavailable testosterone, and possibly decreased sensitivity of the testosterone receptor. The term andropause has been used to describe a syndrome consisting of low libido, osteoporosis, decreased muscle mass, decreased energy and other signs of aging [34].

Differential Diagnosis

The major issue in the treatment of male hypoactive sexual desire disorder is a differential diagnosis between etiologies that are predominantly psychogenic versus those which are predominantly biogenic. Lifelong problems with desire tend to be situational and are presumed to be predominantly psychogenic where acquired global problems may be psychogenic, mixed or organic in etiology. One first attempts to identify treatable causes of low desire such as depression and drug side effects. Most other known causes of biogenic hypoactive sexual desire disorder in males are endocrinological. Common causes include hypogonadism, hyperprolactinemia, and thyroid abnormalities. These disorders tend to be gradual in onset in global. However, a global presentation may appear situational to an unskilled clinician. For example, a man might report low libido with a regular partner yet report increased libido with a novel partner. For these reasons, routine laboratory examinations are recommended in men complaining of acquired, global hypoactive sexual desire disorder. Typically, these laboratory examinations would include thyroid indices, serum prolactin, and serum testosterone. If available, serum free testosterone is preferred. A blood draw before 10:00 AM is recommended as testosterone secretion has diurnal variation. Serum free testosterone is recommended as approximately 80% of circulating testosterone is bound to serum hormone-binding globulin and considered not to be bioavailable. Approximately, 2% occurs as free testosterone and about 20% is loosely bound to albumin.

Conclusions

Hypoactive sexual desire disorders often remain treatment refractory. Considerable effort is being made by pharmaceutical companies to identify effective interventions for female sexual disorders. In hypogonadal men, a number of forms of androgen replacement are available. However, androgen replacement is not without its risks and requires careful monitoring. There is a paucity of evidence-based interventions for psychogenic hypoactive sexual desire disorder in either sex.

References

1 Riley A, May K: Sexual desire disorders; in Gabbard G (ed): Treatment of Psychiatric Disorders, ed 3. Washington DC, American Psychiatric Press, 2001, pp 1849–1872.
2 Masters WH, Johnson VE: Human Sexual Inadequacy. Boston, Mass, Little Brown, 1970.
3 American Psychiatric Association. Diagnostic and Statistical Manual of Mental Disorders. ed 4. Text Revision. Washington DC, American Psychiatric Press, 2000.
4 Maurice W: Male hypoactive sexual desire disorder; in Balon R, Segraves R (eds): Handbook of Sexual Dysfunction. Boca Raton, Fla., Taylor & Francis, 2005, pp 67–110.
5 Segraves R, Woodard T: Female hypoactive sexual desire disorder: history and current status. J Sex Med 2006;3:408–418.
6 Basson R, Leiblum S, Brotto L, derogates L, Fergusion D, Fourcroy J, Fugl-Meyer K, Graziottin A, Heiman J, Lann E, Meston C, Schover L, van Lankveld J, Schultz WW: Revised definitions of women's sexual dysfunction. J Sex Med 2004;1:40–48.
7 Basson R: Female hypoactive sexual desire disorder; in Balon R, Segraves R (eds): Handbook of Sexual Dysfunction. Boca Raton, Florida, Taylor and Francis, 2005, pp 43–66.
8 Laumann E, Nicolosi A, Glasser D, Paik A, Gingell C, Moriera E, Wang T: Sexual problems among women and men aged 40–80 years: prevalence and correlates identified in the Global Study of Sexual Attitudes and Behavior. Int J Impot Res 2005;17:39–57.
9 Eplov L, Giraldi A, Davidsen M, Garde K, Kamper-Jorgensen F: Sexual desire in a nationally representative Danish population. J Sex Med 2006;4:47–56.
10 Dunn K: Satisfaction in the sex life of a general population sample. J Sex Marital Ther 2000;26:141–151.
11 Klusmann D: Sexual motivation and the duration of partnership. Arch Sex Behav 2002;41:275–287.
12 Mercer C, Fenton K, Wellings K, Macdowall W, McManus S, Nanchalal K, Erens B: Sexual function problems and help seeking behavior in Britain: national probability sample survey. Br Med J 2003;327: 426–427.
13 McCabe M: Evaluation of a cognitive behavioral program for people with sexual dysfunction. J Sex Marital Ther 2001;27:259–271.
14 Greenblatt R, Wilcox E: Hormonal therapy of fibromyomas of the uterus. S Surg 1941;10:334–346.
15 Greenblatt R, Barfield W, Garner J, Calk G, Harold J: Evaluation of an estrogen, androgen and estrogen-androgen combination and a placebo in the treatment of the menopause. J Clin Endocrinol 1950; 10:1547–1558.
16 Sherwin B, Gelfand M, Brender W: Androgen enhances sexual motivation in females: a prospective crossover study of sex steroid administration in the surgical menopause. Psychosom Med 1985;47: 339–351.
17 Shifren J, Braustein G, Simon J: Transdermal testosterone treatment in women with impaired sexual function after oopohorectomy. N Engl J Med 2000; 243:682–688.

18 Davis S, Davison SL, Donath S, Bell R: Circulating androgen levels and self-reported sexual function in women. J Am Med Assoc 2005;294:91–96.
19 Long C: A randomized comparative study of the effects of oral and topical estrogen therapy on the vaginal vascularization and sexual function in hysterectomized postmenopausal women. Menopause 2006;13:737–743.
20 Segraves RT, Clayton A, Croft H, Wolf A, Warnock J: Bupropion sustained release for the treatment of hypoactive sexual desire disorder in premenopausal women. J Clin Psychopharmacol 2004;24:339–342.
21 Invernizzi R, Sacchetti G, Parini S, Acconcia S, Samanin R: Flibanserin, a potential antidepressant drug, lowers 5HT and raised dopamine in the rat prefrontal cortex dialysate; role of 5HT (1A) receptors. Br J Pharmacol 2003;139:1281–1288.
22 Diamond L: Co-administration of low dose intranasal PT-141, a melanocortin receptor agonist, and sildenafil to men with erectile dysfunction results in an enhanced erectile response. Urology 2005;65:755–759.
23 McKinlay J, Feldman H: Age-related variation in sexual activity and interest in normal men: results from the Massachusetts Male Aging Study; in Rossi As (ed): Sexuality across the Life Cycle. Chicago, The University of Chicago Press, 1994, pp 261–285.
24 Laumann E, Paik A, Rosen R: Sexual dysfunctions in the United States. J Am Med Assoc 1999;281:537–544.
25 LoPiccolo J: Friedman Broad spectrum treatment of low sexual desire: integration of cognitive, behavioral and systemic therapy; in Leiblum S , Rosen R (eds): Sexual Desire Disorders. New York, Guilford Press, 1988, pp 107–144.
26 Balon R: Depression, antidepressants and human sexuality. Prim Psychiatry 2007;14:42–50.
27 Delgado P, Brannans S, Mallinckrodt C, Tran P, McNamara R, Wang F, Watkin J, Detre M: Sexual functioning assessed in 4 double-blind placebo and paroxetine controlled trials of duloxetine for major depressive disorder. J Clin Psychiatry 2005;66:682–691.
28 Landen M, Eriksson E, Agren H, Fahlen T: Effect of buspirone on sexual function in depressed patients treated with selective serotonin reuptake inhibitors. J Clin Psychopharmacol 1999;192:68–71.
29 Balon R: SSRI-associated sexual dysfunction. Am J Psychiatry 2006;163:1504–1509.
30 Knegtering R, Bruggeman R: What are the effects of antipsychotics on sexual functioning. Prim Psychiatry 2007;14:51–56.
31 Crenshaw T, Goldberg J, Stern W: Pharmacological modification of psychosexual dysfunction. J Sex Marital Ther 1987;13:239–252.
32 Carani C, Isidori A, Granata A, Carosa E, Maggi M, Lenzi A, Jannini E: Multicenter study on the prevalence of sexual symptoms in male hypo-and hyperthyroid patients. J Clin Endocrinol Metab 2005;90:1–15.
33 Gray P, Singh A, Woodhouse L, Storer T, Casaburi R, Dzehov J: Dose-dependent effects of testosterone on sexual function, mood, and visuospatial cognition in older men. J Clin Endocrinol Metab 2005;90:3838–3846.
34 Wespes E, Shulman C: Male andropause, myth, reality and treatment. Int J Impot Res 2002;14 (suppl 1):S93–S98.

R.T. Segraves, MD, PhD
MetroHealth-Psychiatry
2500 MetroHealth Drive
Cleveland, OH 44109 (USA)
Tel. +1 216 7783634, Fax +1 216 7785907, E-Mail rsegraves@metrohealth.org

Balon R (ed): Sexual Dysfunction. The Brain-Body Connection.
Adv Psychosom Med. Basel, Karger, 2008, vol 29, pp 33–49

Erectile Dysfunction

Kevan Wylie

Porterbrook Clinic, Nether Edge Hospital, Sheffield, UK

Abstract

Erectile dysfunction is a common problem affecting sexual function in men. Approximately one in 10 men over the age of 40 is affected by this condition and the incidence is age related. Erectile dysfunction is a sentinel marker for several reversible conditions including peripheral and coronary vascular disease, hypertension and diabetes mellitus. Endothelial dysfunction is a common factor between the disease states. Concurrent conditions such as depression, late-onset hypogonadism, Peyronie's disease and lower urinary tract symptoms may significantly worsen erectile function, other sexual and relationship issues and penis dysmorphophobia. A focused physical examination and baseline laboratory investigations are mandatory. Management consists of initiating modifiable lifestyle changes, psychological and psychosexual/couples interventions and pharmacological and other interventions. In combination and with treatment of concurrent comorbid states, these interventions will often bring about successful resolution of symptoms and avoid the need for surgical interventions.

Erectile dysfunction (ED) is a common condition which is often kept a secret from both partners and health care professions as much as possible. Many therapies are available and with increasing public awareness and social acceptance of such treatments, the condition is more openly discussed in modern society. However, ED is more than a lifestyle or sexual problem and can be an important early sign of more sinister disease.

Definition

ED is defined as persistent or recurrent inability to attain, or to maintain until completion of the sexual activity, an adequate erection; the disturbance causes marked distress or interpersonal difficulties and the ED is not better accounted for by another Axis I disorder (other than a sexual dysfunction) and is not due exclusively to the direct physiological effects of a substance (e.g. a drug of abuse, a medication) or a general medical condition. It should be specified whether this is lifelong type or acquired type, generalized type or situational type and due to psychological factors or due to combined factors.

Epidemiology

ED affects approximately 10% of men in the general population. Worldwide it is estimated that over 100,000,000 men are affected [1]. It is expected that between 1995 and 2025 the prevalence of ED worldwide will have increased by more than 110% [2].

There is a clear age relationship which affects men much more commonly over the age of 40 years with an estimated 30% of men affected between the ages of 40 and 70 [3], and some reports describing over 50% of men over the age of 40 years of age being affected with an incidence approaching 70% by the age of 70 years [4].

Three in 10 men aged between 40 and 80 years of age reported at least one sexual problem. The most frequent problem was early ejaculation (14%) followed by erection difficulties (10%) and problems were found more often with increasing age [5]. A random sample of 1,000 people in different age groups between the ages of 18–75 was selected from 4 diverse general practices in England. With 39% of men and 49% of women responding (1,768 responses in total) the common problems for men were getting an erection (current 21%, lifetime 23%), difficulty maintaining an erection (24 and 25%) and either or both of these (26 and 39%).

The most common presenting problem to UK sexologists from men was ED (70%) [6].

The US national health and social life survey asked questions of 1,410 men and 1,749 women aged between 18 and 59 years [7]. For most questions the response rates did not differ with age except for trouble achieving and maintaining an erection which increased with age in men. The study highlighted that sexual dysfunction was highly associated with unsatisfying personal experiences and relationships.

Erection Processes

Penile erection is described as a neurovascular phenomenon which is influenced by hormonal, biochemical and biomechanical factors both centrally and locally within the penis. The haemodynamics involve increased arterial inflow to the penis, penile blood engorgement and deceased venous outflow. Factors associated with response include corporeal smooth muscle relaxation, venoocclusive function and striated penile muscle activity [8].

It is the contractile state of the corporal smooth muscle cells within the penile vessels and sponge-like trabecular tissue of the corporal-cavernosa and to a lesser extent the corporal-spongiosum that is the fundamental physiological aspect of the erection process. Relaxation of the cells and dilation of the penile blood vessels with expansion of trabecular tissue and subsequent engorgement brings about erection. The finite elastic tunica albuginea ensheathing the dual main corporal bodies of the penis contain the erectile tissue. Blood drainage from the penis through subtunical and emissionary veins are juxtaposed beneath and then transversing the tunica albuginea and are restricted as the penile vessels are compressed and elongated during the hydrological process of penile erection. Secondly, the structural integrity of the erectile tissue is necessary for a normal venoocclusive mechanism. Corporal smooth muscle cells, fibroblasts, collagen, nerves and endothelium contribute towards the mechanism of venoocclusion. The third process of striated penile muscle activity is relevant with the action of the pelvic floor musculature of the bulbospongeosis and ischiocavernosus muscles surrounding the corporal bodies at the base of the penis. Hormonal, central and peripheral neurological control and neurotransmitters all regulate penile erection [9]. The predominant mediator of erection is nitric oxide released from non-adrenergic, non-cholinergic nerve terminations as well as from vascular and sinusoidal endothelium of the penis. Secondary mechanisms modulate this main regulatory control feature including the cholinergic mechanism (parasympathetic control, reducing contractile influence of adrenergic agents such as epinephrine and endothelin-1) and facilitating relaxation by stimulating release of endothelial relaxant substances. These are described in greater detail by Burnett [8].

Secondary messenger molecules are primary intracellular mediators of smooth muscle relaxation – the cyclic nucleotides. These induce tissue relaxation via downstream protein kinase actions which influence ion fluxes within smooth muscle cells. The RhoA/Rho-kinase pathway is another recently identified major intracellular mechanism mediating cavernosal tissue contraction [10].

Aetiology

A number of medical conditions are known to be associated and instrumental in bringing about ED. The commonest group of conditions are those affecting the cardiovascular system and particularly the peripheral vessels. Peripheral vascular disease, hypertension and diabetes mellitus are common conditions in the community and commonly associated with ED. Despite this there has been, until recently, very little research undertaken to establish the relative risk of sexual problems associated with these conditions, predictors and response to intervention and the impact and consequences of the disease state and any treatments provided.

ED and heart disease have both common and shared risk factors. These have been described as diabetes mellitus, hypertension, dyslipidaemia and smoking cigarettes [11–13].

Oxidative stress and damage brings about endothelial dysfunction. Patients with cardiovascular disease and diabetes mellitus share a common factor of endothelial dysfunction. This has been shown to occur prior to the formation of atherosclerotic plaques and provides the link between vascular disease and ED [14]. Patients with no apparent cardiovascular disease or diabetes mellitus have also been found to have impaired endothelial function where there is ED [15].

Hence, it is recognised that ED can act as a sentinel for many underlying medical states but the stigma associated with ED leads to only a minority of cases being brought to the attention of medical professionals. ED is considered to be a harbinger of cardiovascular events in some men and so prompt investigation and intervention for cardiovascular risk factors is imperative [16].

Montorsi et al. [17] provide illustrative representation to show the importance of ED as a predictor for subsequent coronary artery disease. The relative arterial diameters illustrate how a 50% reduction in penile artery flow brings about ED long before similar symptoms emerge from coronary artery symptoms.

Symptoms of depression may be the consequences or aetiology of ED. Many common factors may be etiologically responsible for both depression and ED. The prevalence of depression in men with ED was 25% when compared with men without ED in whom it was 13% [18]. A separate survey of over quarter of a million men with ED found the prevalence of depression to be 11.1% [19].

Other conditions which should be excluded include late-onset hypogonadism, Peyronie's disease and prostatic disease.

The interplay between psychological factors as a consequence and reaction to any physical disease state deserves considerable attention. For example around 1 in 3 patients following a myocardial infarction suffer with symptoms of anxiety and depression [20]. Anxiety and depression have been noted to be major contributors in both the aetiology and maintenance of ED. The psychological impact of incapacity and disability, ongoing circulatory dysfunction with heart failure and the consequences of drug treatment for both cardiovascular diseases as well as for depression can all have a compounding and negative impact on a person's wellbeing, quality of life and erectile function [21].

Communicating with Patients

For those who have the sequelae of cardiovascular disease, such as a myocardial infarction, communication between physicians and patients remains limited [22, 23]. The whole issue of communication and discussion around themes of sexuality with patients remains unclear, although the evidence would suggest that increasingly patients expect to be able to receive clear and accurate information from their physicians, even if it is them who have to raise the subject.

A postal questionnaire sent to doctors, nurses, physiotherapists and occupational therapists investigated views about acute and rehabilitation settings and discussing sexual issues with patients [24]. 90% of respondents agreed that the sexual issue should be addressed, although 68% admitted to never initiating discussion, 26% initiated only a few times and only 6% initiated on a regular basis. The reasons given as barriers to communication were lack of training (76%), lack of time (67%) and embarrassment (50%). Additional attention barriers were patient age (61%), physical status (54%), gender (52%) and marital status (42%). Only 14% reported significant training with the other 86% having either no training (46%) or only minimal (40%). There are certain groups of men whose needs are often neglected including the older man who may be more reluctant to disclose sexual symptoms to a physician [25, 26].

Similar issues of poor training and fear of raising the subject have been described by Humphrey and Nazareth [27] and Rele and Wylie [28]. Humphrey and Nazareth noted personal embarrassment, inadequate skills and knowledge and a fear that 'a flood gate' might be opened were described.

Gott et al. [29] undertook in depth semi-structured interviews of 22 GPs and 35 practice nurses. The barriers they described were 'opening up a can of worms' that would have to have been followed through, fear of patients believing that the clinicians may be sexualising the consultation, middle age and older patients who may be more easily offended and sensitive to such issues, those from ethnic minorities who may not openly discuss such issues, religious beliefs and fear of possible prejudice of non-heterosexual patients as well as a general uncertainty of knowing which terms to use, were all cited as key barriers.

Physical Examination

Generally, the distribution of body hair, adipose tissue and muscle bulk should be recorded. All men should have blood pressure, heart rate, waist circumference and weight measured. Any evidence of abdominal masses can be recorded.

All patients should have a focused physical examination of the genitals. This is essential if there is a rapid onset of pain, deviation of the penis during tumescence, symptoms of hypogonadism or other urological symptoms in the past or current. The genitalia should be inspected and the general size, shape and characteristics of the penis and testicles should be noted. When evidence of fibrosis of the penis (Peyronie's disease) or problems with the foreskin including phimosis and paraphimosis observed, these should be recorded. Testicular size, consistency and presence should be noted. Specific neurological examination includes the glandular pudendal reflex and the cremasteric reflex as well as general sensation in the perineal area.

Where there are genitourinary or protracted secondary ejaculatory symptoms digital prostate examination is advised.

Laboratory Investigations

All patients should be screened for fasting blood glucose to exclude diabetes mellitus. A total testosterone level should be measured between 8:00 am and 10:00 am, and if this is low it should be repeated alongside measures of FSH and LH. A reasonable estimate of free and bioavailable testosterone levels can be calculated from total testosterone, sex hormone-binding globulin and albumin levels. Use of an online calculator may be helpful such as that on the ISSAM website www.issam.ch/freetesto. htm. The serum prolactin should be measured in all cases and if raised should be repeated in a fasting state and cannulated. A fasting lipid profile is useful to assess total cholesterol and HDL levels. Where urological symptoms are evident a PSA level should be measured. If there are concurrent problems of sexual desire then thyroxine/TSH should be measured.

Additional Investigations

The use of intra-cavernosal injection of alprostadil, (a prostaglandin E1) into the corpus cavernosum of the penis to augment penile response either in clinic or during either RigiScan investigation or ultrasound investigation is well reported. The specific use of specialist investigations varies between departments and clinical need. Specialist units may use devices such as the RigiScan which allows both real time (provocative) and night time/sleep (nocturnal) recordings or ultrasound recordings for confirming the diagnosis and extent of primarily vascular disease. However its value in discriminating between neurological and psychogenic disease is also worth of note [see 30]. Where there are suggestions of veno-occlusive disorder, ultrasonography followed by, if necessary, cavernosometry or cavernosography is appropriate [BSSM, in press]. Where patients have symptoms suggestive of significant psychological contribution nocturnal penile tumescence and/or provocative RigiScan may be useful to confirm normal function [31]. The normal parameters would be a minimum of 3 erections per night on at least one of three nights. Each erection should last at least 10 min with change in girth at both the base and the tip and with greater than 60% rigidity at the tip.

Measurement Tools

Validated questionnaires including the International Index of Erection Function (IIEF) [32] and the validated shorter version the Sexual Health Invention for Men (SHIM) can assess sexual function domains as well as the impact of interventions and treatments. They do not replace a through history or medical examination.

The use of the self-administered IIEF questionnaire is the basic tool used in assessing and monitoring treatment in erectile function. It is simple for patients to complete and is sensitive and specific in detecting treatment-related changes in ED. Fifteen questions deal with erectile function, orgasmic function, sexual desire, intercourse satisfaction and overall satisfaction. The ability to maintain erections during sexual intercourse is the best discriminator between men with and without ED. The score of 21 has a sensitivity of 98% and specificity of 88%. Scores of 22 and above indicate normal ED.

Management

Modifiable Factors

Obesity is associated with decreased levels of testosterone and free testosterone and increased peripheral conversion of testosterone and other androgens to oestrogen. Weight loss may therefore influence testosterone levels [33].

A randomised single-blind trial of 110 obese men aged between 35 and 55 years without diabetes, hypertension or hyperlipidemia and who had ED with an IIEF score of 21 or less were assigned to either advice to achieve a loss of 10% or more of their total body weight by reducing calorie intake and increasing physical activity or a control group who were given general information about healthy food choice and exercise. Lifestyle changes were associated with improvement in around one third of obese men with ED at baseline [34].

High body mass index may be related with sleep apnoea which is itself associated with ED. Treatment with continued positive airway pressure to the nasal passages improves erectile function [35].

A recent comprehensive evaluation identified via a Medline search until July 2007 supports the association between metabolic syndrome, ED and low-grade inflammatory state [36]. The increased circulating levels of inflammatory and endothelial-prothrombotic compounds are related to the presence and severity of ED. Specific inflammatory biomarkers and their combination appear to have the potential to aid the diagnosis or exclusion of ED. It is concluded that ED and coronary artery disease may confer a similar unfavourable impact on the inflammatory and prothrombotic state and that ED adds an incremental activation in addition to coronary artery disease. Lifestyle and risk factor modification as well as pharmacological therapy are associated with anti-inflammatory effects.

A Mediterranean style diet has been shown to lead to an improvement of erectile function score (IIEF-5) after 2 years with around one third of men regaining normal erectile function with a significant improvement in endothelial function score and inflammatory markers (hsCRP) [37]. As noted, Esposito [34] reported that the loss of total body weight by greater than 10% and the increase in physical activity led to an improvement in the IIEF-5 score and reduction in serum concentrations of IL-6 and hsCRP after 2 years. The potential role of phosphodiesterase type 5 (PDE5) inhibitors, statins and ACE inhibitors are considered further by Vlachopoulos et al. [36].

Smoking cigarettes increases the risk of cardiovascular disease which in turn is associated with ED. A recent article supports the association between ED and smoking cigarettes [38]. The controversies regarding the association between smoking and ED are considered further in this article. Nicotine is also a potent vasoconstrictor and for those people with compromised arterial function the immediate effect of smoking a cigarette persists for at least 2 h.

The role of illicit substance abuse is a further factor where lifestyle change can have a marked impact on ED. Lifetime use of ED medications was reported as used in a quarter of men surveyed in a substance abuse treatment outpatient clinic [39].

Psychological and Psychosexual Couple Interventions

The role of psychological treatments in conjunction with physical treatments remains an area of controversy and debate. For many men, there is an inevitable psychological cognitive or emotional response to a failure to achieve or maintain a rigid erection which he considers essential to have satisfactory sexual intercourse either alone or with his partner. For some men there may be a wholly psychological contribution towards the ED. In either case, there is often a rejection of the suggestion that engagement in psychological or talking therapies will bring benefit to the man and his partner. For some patients, it is helpful to demonstrate the presence of an adequate erection. This has included the use of a pharmacological induced erection within the clinic (for example using intra-cavernosal alprostadil) or by using other evidence to demonstrate erectile capacity. Use of partner recall can be helpful but in other circumstances objective measurement such as nocturnal RigiScan or ultrasonography demonstrating excellent function is required before the patient agrees to engage in a talking therapy.

The literature is sparse for randomised control trials as the primary or secondary treatment for ED. With this in mind the interested reader is referred to a recent article which reviewed the various psychological and theoretical frameworks and review of literature for the use of talking therapies for ED [40]. A recent Cochrane review of psychosocial interventions for ED [41] found evidence that group therapy improves ED in selected patients who received group therapy, and sildenafil showed significant improvement of ED. Men were less likely than those receiving only sildenafil to drop out.

Pharmacological and Other Interventions

First-Line Oral Agents

Three potential selective PDE5 inhibitors are currently licensed with proven efficacy and safety.

Sildenafil licensed in 1998 is effective within 30–60 min of oral ingestion. Efficacy is reduced after a heavy fatty meal. The recommended starting dose is 50 mg adapted to the patient's response and side effects. Nightly low-dose sildenafil may improve recovery of erectile function after nerve sparing radical prostatectomy [42]. In a subgroup of patients PDE6 receptors are inhibited in the rods of the retina leading to a blue hue, but this is unlikely to affect common visual tasks [43].

Tadalafil may become effective within 30 min of ingestion but it is often necessary to advise ingestion 2 h before anticipated activity with efficacy then maintained for up to 36 h. Efficacy is not much influenced by food. Patients are advised to start at 10 mg and increase the dose to 20 mg depending on response and side effects.

Vardenafil is effective within 30 min of oral ingestion. Effect is reduced by heavy fatty meals. There is evidence that in specific populations vardenafil has been shown to be superior to placebo. These have included studies of men with hypertension with meta-analysis of clinical trial data [44], renal transplant recipients [45] and men with ED caused by spinal cord injury [46]. Vardenafil has been shown to have an extended duration of efficacy of up to 8 h post-dose for some patients [47].

The interested reader is referred to recent articles which provide much greater detail about these agents [48, 49]. The PDE5 inhibitors have been confirmed as a valuable treatment option for ED in men with diabetes mellitus [50]. Data would not suggest any relationship between nonarteritic anterior ischemic optic neuropathy in men who take sildenafil for ED [51].

A new treatment satisfaction scale which is a brief comprehensive self-report measure of patient and partner satisfaction has recently been utilised in studies and reported as a potential product for evaluating 'treatment effectiveness' by measuring more general treatment satisfaction for men with ED and their partners [52].

Choice or Preference between PDE5 Inhibitors

Many patients will show preference to the response to one or more of these agents. There is much individual variation regarding onset and efficacy as well as duration of onset. Side effects may also influence patient continuation.

Several concerns regarding studies of preference of PDE5 inhibitors which have been published arise due to questionable study design or bias selection. Eardley et al. [53] showed a patient preference for tadalafil (71%) versus sildenafil (29%) in an open-label cross-over study of naïve patients for 8 weeks of dose optimisation followed by 4 weeks of assessment. The major reason for the preference was the ability to get an erection long after taking the drug despite similar efficacy. Rubio-Aurioles et al. [54] compared vardenafil with sildenafil in a double-blind cross-over study using fixed doses of 20 mg vardenafil versus 100 mg of sildenafil in non-naïve patients. 38.9% showed a preference to vardenafil compared to 34.5% for tadalafil with 26.6% expressing no preference with similar efficacy. A third study by Tolra et al. [55] compared all three PDE5 inhibitors in an open-label study in treatment-naïve patients. 52% reported favouring tadalafil, 28% sildenafil and 20% vardenafil with the possibility of an erection well after taking the drug being the main reason of preference.

Efficacy rates and adverse events are similar for all three drugs but discontinuation rates were somewhat lower for sildenafil in a review of all randomised trials identified by mid-2005 [56].

Specific Patient Groups

The danger of the combination of PDE5 inhibitors with nitrates is well established – they must not be combined because of the marked risk of hypotension. This is regardless of the preparation type such as nitroglycerin, isosorbide mononitrate or isosorbide dinitrate. Nicorandil and recreational drugs such as amyl nitrate (poppers) also contain nitrates. Catastrophic hypotension can occur.

The majority of men with coronary heart disease are able to safely resume sexual activity and use ED therapies following myocardial infarction. Contraindications would be men who continue to have unstable cardiac states, recent myocardial infarction (within 6 months) unstable dysrhythmias or heart failure. The Princeton consensus group have stated that 'a man with ED and no cardiac symptoms is a cardiac patient unless proven otherwise'. They go on to differentiate cardiac risk as low – which should be managed in primary care, intermediate – which can be dealt with in primary or secondary care, and those in high cardiac risk who should not be offered treatment for ED in primary care. The full recommendations are available in the consensus document [16].

Alpha-blockers interact with the PDE5 inhibitors resulting in orthostatic hypotension. The UK SPC does not recommend the use of tadalafil with alpha-blockers. Vardenafil should be initiated at the lowest dose with patients stabilised on alpha-blocker therapy with the two drugs separated by 6 h (except with tamsulosin in which case vardenafil can be used at any time). Sildenafil should be initiated on the lowest dose in patients stabilised on alpha-blocker therapy separating dosing by at least 4 h.

Padma-Nathan et al. [57] reported that 75 patients who commenced on 50–100 mg for 4 weeks after nerve sparing surgery and continuing thereafter for 36 weeks found 27% retained normal function without the need for therapy compared to 4% in the placebo group in patients who had radical prostatectomy and frequent dosing thereafter to preserve erectile function following surgery. The benefit to this group of patients is the reduced need for prolonged treatment.

The management of sexual dysfunction and in particular erection difficulties for patients prescribed anti-depressant medication has been reviewed by Lisa et al. [58]. Adding sildenafil had more effect than placebo in treating antidepressant-induced ED in three studies.

Second-Line Therapies

Second-line therapies include intra-cavernosal injections of alprostadil, papaverine or VIP/phentolamine, intraurethral alprosadil (MUSE) and vacuum constriction devices. The latter may be as effective as intra-cavernosal injection alprostadil at increasing rigidity but are less effective for orgasm and may block ejaculation [59].

One side effect of intra-cavernosal and inter-urethral alprostadil is prolonged erection (priapism). If this process occurs for greater than 4 h erection must be reduced to avoid potential complications or permanent ED. Aspiration and sometimes injection of phenylepherine are necessary [48]. Surgical intervention and rarely penile prosthesis are required.

Third-Line Therapies

Where prosthesis are required a choice of malleable (semi-rigid) or inflatable (two or three piece) are available. Fewer mechanical complications and simpler implantation technique gives preference to the two piece inflatable prosthesis [48]. Concurrent ED treatments are often necessary and valuable, e.g. to attend to the 'soft glans' phenomenon. Vascular surgery is occasionally indicated in young men with a history of pelvic trauma.

A recent search in appraisal of RCTs by clinical evidence [59] considered the treatment for ED to be beneficial by the use of intra-urethral and intra-cavernosal alprostadil, apomorphine and the PDE5 inhibitors sildenafil, tadalafil and vardenafil. Those considered likely to be beneficial include Ginseng, penile prosthesis, psychosexual counselling, vacuum devices and yohimbine. Topical alprostadil and papaverine either alone or in combination with phentolomine and/or alprostadil had a trade off between benefits and harm. Cognitive behavioural therapy was found to have unknown effectiveness. The PDE5 inhibitors have as their main contra-indicator concomitant use of nitrates due to the association with severe hypotension and death. Intra-cavernosal and intra-urethral alprostadil and papaverine may cause penile pain in up to 40% of men. Vacuum devices may be as effective as intra-cavernosal alprostadil at increasing rigidity but less effective for orgasm and may block ejaculation. Psychosexual counselling and cognitive behavioural therapy may improve sexual function in men with psychological ED but few good quality studies have been found.

Comorbidity

Late-Onset Hypogonadism

The Endocrine Society of North America recommends that testosterone therapy is offered to men with ED who have unequivocally low testosterone levels after evaluation of possible courses of ED and consideration of established therapies for ED [60].

Zitzmann et al. [61] report an increasing likelihood of symptoms with a decrease in the concentration of androgens. Although these are not absolute, it provides a novel way of understanding the various symptoms which vary with different testosterone levels and so potentially the subsequent response to any replacement therapy. ED correlates with very low levels of androgen concentrations.

Treatment with testosterone alone is sufficient for a number of patients including elderly men with sexual problems [62]. Bolona et al. [63] review the inconsistence and unexplainable results across clinical trials with wide confidence intervals and possible reporting bias.

The evidence for combining testosterone and PDE5 inhibitors is reviewed by Greco et al. [64] and Saad et al. [65]. The presence of venoocclusive dysfunction due to testosterone insufficiency strengthens the need to augment sildenafil with testosterone as an adjunctive therapy, particularly in those who do not respond to sildenafil alone [66].

The concern that testosterone causes prostate cancer development and growth has been reviewed by Morgentaler [67]. There is no evidence of this and the contraindication of testosterone replacement in men following, for example, radical prostatectomy for prostate cancer will now need fresh evaluation.

A recent summary by Traish and Guay [68] proposes that androgens regulate multiple signalling pathways and the structure of cavernosal tissue and cellular components within the corpus cavernosa. The mechanisms include regulation of NOS isoform expression and activity, regulation of PDE5 expression and activity, regulation of the alpha-adrenoceptor expression and function, regulation of smooth muscle cell growth and response to vasodilators, regulation of connective tissue metabolism and deposition of ECM, regulation of differentiation of progenitor vascular/stroma cells into myogenic and adipogenic lineages and maintaining neural structure and function.

Testosterone may have a protective role in the development of metabolic syndrome and subsequent diabetes mellitus and cardiovascular disease in aging men. However clinical trials on ED need to confirm this assumption [69].

Peyronie's Disease

This condition often presents as ED alone without the full triad of symptoms of ED, bend of the penis and pain in the penis shaft. As such it must be attended to where clinically indicated.

Lower Urinary Tract Symptoms

Lower urinary tract symptoms (LUTS) and ED are associated independently of age and major co-morbidities and vascular risk factors may be a common link. Medical and surgical treatment options for LUTS often impact on erectile and other sexual function selection of PDE5 inhibitor therapy and specific alpha-1 blockers should be considered [70].

Other Sexual and Relationship Issues

Sexual problems may coincide with ED and as such may need treatment in their own right. For example rapid ejaculation or painful intercourse secondary to menopausal changes. There is evidence that women are affected by their partners ED and that ED treatment may have subsequent beneficial effects for the woman [71].

Small Penis Syndrome

This condition, often a part of body dysmorphophobia, should be identified if present as it often results in a failure to respond to conventional treatments [72].

Management of PDE5 Inhibitor Failures

Many patients have high expectations of vardenafil, sildenafil and tadalafil including restoration of sexual response akin to adolescence years. These unrealistic expectations and many other factors may lead to considerable disappointment for patients where sildenafil (and other PDE5 inhibitors) is ineffective. The effectiveness of these agents is not the only factor which is influencing repeat use of the agent. In one study only 69% of those who were successful had a repeat prescription within 6 months [73]. Kendirci et al. [74] have differentiated sildenafil failure in the treatment of erection dysfunction as inter-physician, patient, partner, disease and drug factors.

Certain physician factors may be modifiable including issues of inadequate information and instruction about dose variation at onset which has been identified as potentially valuable in helping patients with ED who have previously failed treatment with the drug [75]. The level of understanding and proficiency of the treating physician, the time spent educating the patient, lack of problem follow up and re education, lack of involvement and the education of the partner are also important factors.

The quality of non-sexual aspects of the relationship should not be underestimated. A paradigm of combined therapy has been developed by Althof [76].

A number of approaches have been suggested in the management of PDE5 inhibitor failures including optimisation of treatment with an adequate number of attempts and proper dose titration as well as attending to issues such as: partner sexual dysfunction and limited sex education; modification of risk factors including lifestyle changes, smoking cessation, lipid optimisation, reduced alcohol ingestion, increasing exercise, reducing obesity and substitution of offending mediations; switch to other oral medications; daily use of sildenafil; switching to other ED treatments such as vacuum devices, intra-urethral or intra-cavernosal alprostadil or use of combination therapies including attending to other co morbidities [77–81].

The probability of successful intercourse will increase after each attempt until an eventual plateau is reached [82]. In one study, success at first attempt was 54%, increasing to 64% at second attempt, and reached an eventual plateau of 86%. Informing patients that up to 8 attempts may be required to achieve intercourse especially if they have been sexually inactive and are likely to be anxious during the first few attempts can be helpful. High doses beyond recommended doses have been described but are associated with higher rates of side effects.

Daily use in patients with vascular ED who had a nightly intake of 50 mg of sildenafil compared to those who used it on a as needed basis were shown to have improved cavernosal blood flow during pharmacologically induced erections and Doppler investigation [83]. In a study with men having undergone nerve-sparing radical prostatectomy the authors documented an increase in cavernosal smooth muscle content [84].

Future Developments

The introduction of transfer of genetic material into human cells to either supplement normal cellular function or restore defective function is the basis of gene therapy which may well become a treatment for ED in the future [85]. Other emerging treatments include the use of pelvis floor exercise [86] and the novel use of agents such as cabergoline [87] for psychogenic ED.

Conclusions

ED serves as a sentinel marker for more serious cardiovascular and psychosocial problems. Clinicians should make enquiry about the condition regardless of specialty. Where identified, aetiology should be established and treatment options outlined. The aim is restoration of erectile function within a sexual situation which is desirable and comfortable for the man and his partner.

References

1 Russell ST, Khandheria B, Nehra A: Erectile Dysfunction and Cardiovascular Disease. Mayo Clin Proc 2004;79:782–794.

2 Haczynksi J, Lew-Starowicz Z, Darewicz B, Krajka K, Piotrowicz R, Ciesielska B: The prevalence of erectile dysfunction in men visiting out patient clinics. Int J Impot Res 2006;18:359–363.

3 DeBusk R, Drory Y, Goldstein I, Jackson G, Kaul S: Management of sexual dysfunction in patients with cardiovascular disease: Recommendations of the Princeton Consensus Panel. Am J Cardiol 2000;86: 2, 175–181.

4 Seidman SN: Exploring the relationship between depression and erectile dysfunction in aging men. J Clin Psychiatry 2002;63:5, 5–12.

5 Nicolosi A, et al: Sexual behaviour and sexual dysfunctions after age 40: the global study of sexual attitudes and behaviours. J Urol 2004;64:991–997.

6 Wylie KR, DeColomby P, Giami A: Sexology as a profession in the United Kingdom. Int J Clin Pract 2004;58:764–768.

7 Laumann EO, Paik A, Rosen RC: Sexual dysfunction in the United States: prevalence and predictors. JAMA 1999;281:537–544.

8 Burnett AL: Erectile dysfunction; science and medicine. Annu Rev Sex Res 2006;17:101–115.

9 Sáenz de Tejada, Angulo J, Cellek S, González-Cadavid N, Heaton J, Pickard R, Simonsen U: Physiology of erectile function. J Sex Med 2004;1: 254–265.

10 Jin L, Burnett AL: RhoA/Rho-kinase in erectile tissue: mechanisms of disease and therapeutic insights. Clin Sci 2006;110:153–165.

11 Schwarz ER, Rastogi S, Kapur V, Sulemanjee N, Rodriquez JJ: Erectile dysfunction in heart failure patients. J Am Coll Cardiol 2006;48:6, 1111–1119.

12 Vacanti L, Caramelli B: Distress: Associated variables of erectile dysfunction post acute myocardial infarction. Pilot study. Int J Impot Res 2005;17: 204–206.

13 Gazzaruso C, Giordanetti S, DeAmici E, Bertone G, Falcone C, Geroldi D, Fratino P, Solerte SB, Garzaniti A: Relationship between erectile dysfunction and silent myocardial ischemia in apparently uncomplicated type 2 diabetic patients. Circulation 2004; 110:22–26.
14 Wang BC, Cunningham G, Dobs A, Iranmanesh A: Is atherosclerotic cardiovascular disease an endocrinological disorder? J Clin Endocrinol Metab 2004; 89:2085–2098.
15 Barrett-Connor E, Goodman-Gruen D, Patay P: Endogenous sex hormones and cognitive function in older men. J Clin Endocrinol Metab 1999;84: 3681–3685.
16 Kostis JB, Jackson G, Rosen R, Barrett-Connor E, Billups K, Burnett AL, Carson C 3rd, Cheitlin M, Debusk R, Fonseca V, Ganz P, Goldstein I, Guay A, Hatzichristou D, Hollander JE, Hutter A, Katz S, Kloner RA, Mittleman M, Montorsi F, Montorsi P, Nehra A, Sadovsky R, Shabsigh R: Sexual dysfunction and cardiac risk (the Second Princeton Consensus Conference). Am J Cardiol 2005;96:313–321.
17 Montorsi P: Is erectile dysfunction the 'tip of the iceberg' of a systemic vascular disorder? Eur Urol 2003;44:3, 352.
18 Carani C, Isidori A, Granata A: Multicenter study on the prevalence of sexual symptoms in male hypo- and hyperthyroid patients. J Endocrinol Clin Metab 2005;90:6472–6479.
19 Seftel A, Sun P, Swindle R: The prevalence of hypertension, hyperlipidemia, diabetes mellitus and depression in men with erectile dysfunction. J Urol 2004; 171:2341–2345.
20 Boersma SN, Maes S, van Elderen T: Goal disturbance predicts health-related quality of life and depression four months after myocardial infarction. Br J Health Psychol 2005;10:615–630.
21 Rastogi S, Rodriguez JJ, Kapur V, Schwarz ER: Why do patients with heart failure suffer from erectile dysfunction? A critical review and suggestions on how to approach this problem. Int J Impot Res 2005; 17:S25–S36.
22 Soloman H, DeBusk R, Jackson G: Erectile dysfunction: the need to be evaluated, the right to be treated. Am Heart J 2005;150:4, 620–626.
23 Rerkpattanapipat P, Stanek MS, Kotler MN: Sex and the heart: what is the role of the cardiologist? Eur Heart J 2001;22:3, 201–208.
24 Haboubi NHJ, Lincoln N: Views of health professionals on discussing sexual issues with patients. Disabil Rehabil 2003;25:291–296.
25 Enzlin P, Mak R, Kittel F, Demyttenaere K: Sexual functioning in a population-based study of men aged 40–69 years: the good news. Int J Impot Res 2004;16:512–520.
26 Lindau ST, Schumm LP, Laumann EO, Levinson W, O'Muircheartaigh CA, Waite LJ: A study of sexuality and health among older adults in the United States. N Engl J Med 2007;357:762–774.
27 Humphrey S, Nazareth I: GP's views on their management of sexual dysfunction. Fam Pract 2001;18: 516–518.
28 Rele K, Wylie K: Management of psychosexual and relationship problems in general mental health services by psychiatry trainees. Int J Clin Pract 2007; 61:10, 1701–1704.
29 Gott M, Galena E, Hinchliffe S, Elford H: 'Opening a Can of Worms': GP and practice nurse barriers to talking about sexual health in Primary Care. Fam Pract 2004;21:5, 528–536.
30 Wylie KR, Davies-South D, Steward D, Walters S, Iqbal M, Ryles SA: comparison between portable ultrasound (MIDUS) and nocturnal RigiScan when confirming the diagnosis of vascular organic erectile disorder. Int J Impot Res 2006;18:354–358.
31 Wylie KR, Hallam-Jones R, Perrett A: Some of the potential implications of integrated assessment for male erectile disorder. Sex Marital Ther 1999;14: 359–369.
32 Rosen RC, et al: The International Index of Erectile Dysfunction (IIEF): a multidimensional scale for assessment of erectile dysfunction. J Urol 1997;49: 822–830.
33 Sharne DH: Erectile dysfunction in obese men (letter). JAMA 2004;292:2467.
34 Esposito K, Marfella R, Ciotola M, Palo C, Giugliano F, Giugliano G, D'Armiento M, D'Andrea F, Giugliano D. Effect of a mediterranean-style diet on endothelial dysfunction and markers of vascular inflammation in the metabolic syndrome. JAMA 2004;292:1440–1446.
35 Perimenis P, Karkoulias K, Markou S, Gyftopoulos K, Athanasopoulos A, Barbalias G, Kiriazopoulou V, Spiropoulos K: The efficacy of sildenafil and continuous positive airway pressure. Int J Importance Res 2004;16:256–260.
36 Vlachopoulos C, Rokkas K, Ioakeimidis N, Stefanadis C: Inflammation, metabolic syndrome, erectile dysfunction, and coronary artery disease: common links. Eur Urol 2007;52:1590–1600.
37 Esposito K, Ciotola M, Giugliano F, De Sio M, Giugliano G, D'Armiento M, Giugliano D: Mediterrean diet improves erectile function in subjects with the metabolic syndrome. Int J Impot Res 2006; 18:405–410.
38 Lam TH, Adbullah ASM, Ho LM, Yip AWC, Fan S: Smoking and sexual dysfunction in Chinese males: findings from men's health survey. Int J Impot Res 2006;18:364–369.

39 Horvath KJ, Calsyn DA, Terry C, Cotton A: Erectile dysfunction medication use among men seeking substance abuse treatment. J Addict Disord 2007;26: 7–13.
40 Wylie K, Machin A: Erectile dysfunction. Prim Psychiatry 2007;14:2, 65–71.
41 Melnik T, Soares BGO, Nasselo AG: Psychosocial interventions for erectile dysfunction. Cochrane Database Syst Rev 2007. Art. No.: CD004825. DOI: 10.1002/14651858.CD004825.pub2.
42 Bannowsky A, Hautmann S, Wefer B, Schulze H, Van der Horst C, Seif C, Braun PM, Juenemann KP: Nightly low-dose sildenafil improves recovery of erectile function after nerve-sparing radical prostatectomy. Eur Urol Suppl 2006;5:141.
43 Stockman A, Sharpe LT, Tufail PD, Kell C, Ripamonti C, Jeffery G: The effect of sildenafil citrate Viagra on visual sensitivity. J vis 2007;7:4.
44 Shabsigh R, Duval S, Shah M, Regan TS, Juhasz M, Veltry LG: Efficacy of vardenafil for the treatment of erectile dysfunction in men with hypertension: a meta-analysis of clinical trial data. Curr Med Res Opin 2007;23:10, 2453–2460.
45 Demir E, Balal M, Paydas S, Sertdemir Y, Erken U: Efficacy and safety of vardenafil in renal transplant recipients with erectile dysfunction. Transplant Proc 2006;38:1379–1381.
46 Giuliano F, Rubio-Aurioles E, Kennelly M, Montorsi F, Kim ED, Finkbeiner AE, Pommerville PJ, Colopy MW, Wilkins HJ, Wachs BH, for the Vardenafil Study Group: Efficacy and safety of vardenafil in men with erectile dysfunction caused by spinal cord injury. Am Acad Neurol 2006;66:210–216.
47 Porst H, Sharlip ID, Hatzichristou D, Rubio-Aurioles E, Gittelman M, Stancil B, Smith PM, Wilkins HJ, Pommerville P: Extended duration of efficacy of vardenafil when taken 8 hours before intercourse: a randomised, double-blind, placebo-controlled study. J Eur Urol 2006;50:1086–1095.
48 Wespes E, Amar E, Hatzichristou D, Hatzimouratidis K, Montorsi F, Pryor J, Vardi Y, EAU: EAU Guidelines on erectile dysfunction: an update. Eur Urol 2006;49:806–815.
49 Wylie KR, MacInnes I: Erectile Dysfunction; in Balon R, Segraves T (eds): Handbook of sexual dysfunction. Boca Raton, Taylor & Francis, 2005.
50 Vardi M, Nini A: Phosphodiesterase inhibitors for erectile dysfunction in patients with diabetes mellitus. Cochrane Database Syst Rev 2007. Art. No.: CD002187. DOI: 10.1002/14651858.CD002187.pub3.
51 Gorkin L, Hvidsten K, Sobel RE, Siegel R: Sildenafil citrate use and the incidence of nonarteritic anterior ischemic optic neuropathy. Int J Clin Pract 2006;60: 500–503.
52 Rosen R, Goldstein I, Huang X, Bangerter K, Taylor T: The Treatment Satisfaction Scale (TTS) is a sensitive measure of treatment effectiveness for both patients and partners: results of a randomised controlled trial with vardenafil. Int Soc Sex Med 2007; 4:1009–1021.
53 Eardley I, Mirone V, Montorsi F, Ralph D, Kell P, Warner MR, Zhao Y, Beardsworth A: An open-label, multicentre, randomized, crossover study comparing sildenafil citrate and tadalafil for treating erectile dysfunction in men naïve to phosphodiesterase 5 inhibitor therapy. BJU Int 2005;96:1323–1332.
54 Rubio-Aurioles E, Porst H, Eardley I, Goldstein I: Comparing vardenafil and sildenafil in the treatment of men with erectile dysfunction and risk factors for cardiovascular disease: a randomized, double-blind, pooled crossover study. J Sex Med 2006;3:1037–1049.
55 Tolrà JR, Campaña JMC, Ciutat LF, Miranda EF: Prospective, randomized, open-label, fixed-dose, crossover study to establish preference of patients with erectile dysfunction after taking the three PDE-5 inhibitors. J Sex Med 2006;3:901–909.
56 Moore RA, Derry S, McQuay HJ: Indirect comparison of interventions using published randomised trials: systematic review of PDE-5 inhibitors for erectile dysfunction. BMC Urol 2005;5:18.
57 Padma-Nathan H, Stecher VJ, Sweeney M, Orazem J, Tseng LJ, Deriesthal H: Minimal time to successful intercourse after sildenafil citrate: results of a randomized, double-blind, placebo-controlled trial. Urology 2003;62:400–403.
58 Lisa R, Taylor M, Hawton K: Strategies for managing sexual dysfunction induced by antidepressant medication. Cochrane Database Syst Rev 2004. Art. No.:CD003382. DOI: 10.1002/ 14651858.CD0033 82.pub2.
59 Tharyan P, Gobalakrishanan G: Erectile dysfunction. Clin Evid 2006;15:1–24.
60 Bhasin S, Cunningham GR, Hayes FJ, Matsumoto AM, Snyder PJ, Swerdloff RS, Montori VM: Testosterone therapy in adult men with androgen deficiency syndromes: an endocrine society clinical practice guideline. J Clin Endocrinol Metab 2006; 91:6, 1995–2010.
61 Zitzmann M, Depenbusch M, Gromoll J, Nieschlag E: Prostate volume and growth in testosterone-substituted hypogonadal men are dependent on the CAG repeat polymorphism of the androgen receptor gene: a longitudinal pharmacogenetic study. J Clin Endocrinol Metab 2003;88:5, 2049–2054.
62 Yassin AA, Saad F: Treatment of sexual dysfunction of hypogonadal patients with long-acting testosterone undecanoate. Asian J Androl 2006;8:3–9.

63 Bolona E, Uraga M, Haddad R, Tracz M, Sideras K, Kennedy CC, Caples S, Erwin P, Montori VM: Testosterone use in men with sexual dysfunction: a systematic review and meta-analysis of randomized placebo-controlled trials. Mayo Clin Proc 2007;82: 20–28.
64 Greco E, Spera G, Aversa A: Combining testosterone and PDE5 inhibitors in erectile dysfunction: basic rationale and clinical evidences. Eur Urol 2006;50:940–947.
65 Saad F, Grahl AS, Aversa A, Yassin AA, Kadioglu A, Moncada I, Eardley I: Effects of testosterone on erectile function: implications for the therapy of erectile dysfunction. BJU Int 2007;99:988–992.
66 Yassin AA, Saad F, Traish A: Testosterone undecanoate restores erectile function in a subset of patients with venous leakage: a series of case reports. J Sex Med2006;3:727–735.
67 Morgentaler A: Testosterone and prostate cancer: an historical perspective on a modern myth. Eur Urol 2006;50:935–939.
68 Traish AM, Guay AT: Are androgens critical for penile erections in humans? Examining the clinical and preclinical evidence. J Sex Med 2006; 3:382–407.
69 Svartberg J: Epidemiology: testosterone and the metabolic syndrome. Int J Impot Res 2007;19:124–128.
70 Ponholzer A, Madersbacher S: Lower urinary tract symptoms and erectile dysfunction; links for diagnosis, management and treatment. Int J Impot Res 2007;19:544–550.
71 Cameron A, Tomlin M: The effect of male erectile dysfunction on the psychosocial, relationship, and sexual characteristics of heterosexual women in the United States. J Sex Martial Ther 2007;33: 135–149.
72 Wylie KR, Eardley I: Penile size and the 'small penis syndrome'. BJUI 2007;1449–1455.
73 Klotz T, Mathers M, Klotz R, Sommer F: Why do patients with erectile dysfunction abandon effective therapy with Sildenafil? Int J Impot Res 2005;17: 2–4.
74 Kendirci M, Tanriverdi O, Trost L, Hellstrom WJ: Management of sildenafil treatment failures. Curr Opin Urol 2006;16:449–459.
75 Gruenwald I, Shenfeld O, Chen J, Raviv G, Richter S, Cohen A, Vardi Y: Positive effect of counselling and dose adjustment in patients with erectile dysfunction who failed treatment with sildenafil. Eur Urol 2006;50:134–140.
76 Althof SE: Sex therapy in the age of pharmacotherapy. Annu Rev Sex Res 2006.
77 McVary KT: Smoking and erectile dysfunction: evidence best analysis. J Urol 2001;166:1624–1632.
78 Shirir R, Koskimäki J, Hakama M, Häkkinen J: Effective lifestyle factors on incidents of erectile dysfunction. Int J Impot Res 2004;16:389–394.
79 Eposito K: Effective lifestyle changes on erectile dysfunction in obese men. A randomised controlled trial. JAMA 2004;291:2978–2904.
80 Nikoobakht M, Nasseh H, Pourkasmaee M: The relationship between lipid profile and erectile dysfunction. Int Importance Res 2005;17:523–526.
81 Rizvi K, Hampson JP, Harvey JN: Do lipid-lowering drugs cause erectile dysfunction? A systematic review. Fam Pract 2002;19:95–98.
82 McCullough AR, Barada JH, Fawzy A, Guay AT, Hatzichristou D: Achieving treatment optimization with sildenafil citrate (Viagra) in patients with erectile dysfunction. J Urol 2002;60:28–38.
83 Sommer F, Schulze W: Treating erectile dysfunction by endotherlial rehabilitation with PDE5 inhibitors. World J Urol 2005;23:385–392.
84 Schwartz EJ, Wong P, Graydon RJ: Sildenafil preserves intracorporeal smooth muscle after radical retropubic prostatectomy. J Urol 2004;171:771–774.
85 Kendirci M, Teloken P, Champion H, Hellstrom W, Bivalacqua T: Gene therapy for erectile dysfunction: fact or fiction? Eur Urol 2006;50:1208–1222.
86 Rosenbaum TY: Pelvic floor involvement in male and female sexual dysfunction and the role of pelvic floor rehabilitation in treatment: a literature review. J Sex Med 2007;4:4–13.
87 Nickel M, Moleda D, Loew T, Rother W, Gil FP: Cabergoline treatment in men with psychogenic erectile dysfunction: a randomised, double-blind, placebo-controlled study. Int J Importance Res 2007; 19:104–107.

Dr. Kevan R. Wylie
Porterbrook Clinic, Nether Edge Hospital
75 Osborne Road
Sheffield S11 9BF (UK)
Tel. +44 114 271 8674, Fax +44 1629 872688, E-Mail k.r.wylie@sheffield.ac.uk

Balon R (ed): Sexual Dysfunction. The Brain-Body Connection.
Adv Psychosom Med. Basel, Karger, 2008, vol 29, pp 50–69

Recent Advances in the Classification, Neurobiology and Treatment of Premature Ejaculation

Marcel D. Waldinger

Department of Psychiatry and Neurosexology, HagaHospital Leyenburg, The Hague, and Department of Psychopharmacology, Faculty of Pharmaceutical Sciences and Rudolf Magnus Institute for Neurosciences, Utrecht University, Utrecht, The Netherlands

Abstract

Premature ejaculation (PE) is distinguished as a 'complaint' versus a 'syndrome'. Complaints of PE in men with normal ejaculation time durations are highly prevalent among the general male population. However, PE syndromes characterized by a rigid pattern of very short ejaculation times have a much lower prevalence. A major insufficiency of the DSM-IV-TR definition of PE is the absence of a cut-off point of its short ejaculation time criterion. Recently, a new classification of PE has been proposed for the pending DSM-V. It has been proposed to distinguish four PE categories; lifelong PE, acquired PE, natural variable PE and premature-like ejaculatory dysfunction. The syndromes differ in ejaculation time duration, frequency and pattern of PE complaints, and its course in life. The difference in underlying pathophysiology and etiology of the different syndromes determines the first choice of treatment. Lifelong PE need to be treated by medication, acquired PE by treatment of its medical cause, medication or psychotherapy. Psychoeducation and reassurance is indicated for men with natural variable PE. Finally, psychotherapy and/or counselling is the first choice of treatment of men with premature-like ejaculatory dysfunction.

Since its first description in medical literature in 1887, premature ejaculation (PE) has given rise to various and sometimes highly contrasting theories, approaches, and treatments [1]. Although PE was initially considered as nothing more than a peculiar anomaly, it was believed to be mainly a psychological disorder for the first half of the 20th century [2]. After the first psychoanalytic publications of Sandor Ferenczi and Karl Abraham in 1908 and 1917, respectively, PE was regarded as a symptom of a neurosis that had to be treated by psychoanalysis in order to solve the unconscious conflicts that were assumed to have caused the neurosis. This purely psychoanalytical explanation was later challenged by Bernhard Schapiro, a German endocrinologist, who in 1943 postulated that PE was not a neurotic but a psychosomatic disorder. He argued that both biological and psychological factors contributed to rapid ejaculatory performances. Years ahead of this time, Schapiro advocated drug treatment in the form of anesthetic ointments to delay ejaculation. In addition, he is credited with identifying the two types of PE recognized today as primary (lifelong) and secondary (acquired) PE. Because he was the first clinician to use a medical approach to PE, Bernhard Schapiro should be regarded as a pioneer in researching this condition. Unfortunately, the accurate differential diagnosis and biological components of Schapiro's arguments were ignored in his time. Psychoanalytic treatment, mainly conducted by psychiatrists, prevailed throughout the 1940s and 1950s, but unfortunately, very little information of this treatment is documented in the literature. However, in 1970 William Masters and Virginia Johnson argued that PE was the result of self-learned behavior and stated that behavioral treatment in the form of the so called squeeze technique could cure in the majority of cases [3]. Their treatment was a modification to the stop-start technique, a masturbation technique, described in 1956 for the first time by James Semans, an English urologist. However, there is a paucity of evidence-based studies demonstrating hard data of its efficacy to delay ejaculation time [2]. In the mid-1990s, the introduction of the selective serotonin reuptake inhibitors (SSRIs) brought about a revolutionary change in the understanding and treatment of PE [1]. Their efficacy in delaying ejaculation together with the increasing interest of neuroscientists, in investigating sexual behavior in laboratory rats led to the end of the supremacy of the behavioristic approach of PE and marked the beginning of the neurobiological view and drug treatment approach. Animal studies and the use of stop-watch assessment of the intravaginal ejaculation latency time (IELT) [4] both during the baseline period and during drug treatment let to a more evidence-based approach of drug treatment trials. Interestingly, during the 1990s and around the millennium the evidence-based methodology to investigate the efficacy of drug treatments of PE has been developed by clinical researchers independently of the pharmaceutical industry as in the 1990s SSRI manufacturers have not been interested in official registration of SSRIs for the treatment of PE [5]. However, this very important period in the history of academic interest in PE ended in 2004 when some pharmaceutical companies became interested in PE. In a short period of time, their studies and publications on PE have given rise to fierce debate in sexual medical literature on how PE should defined, which methodology and statistics should be used to measure drug treatment efficacy, and which treatment should be regarded as optimal to treat PE with regard to efficacy, side effects and noninterferences with spontaneity of sexual performance [6, 7].

Classification

Complaint versus Disorder

A major misconception in the literature on PE is the idea that PE always represents a male sexual 'disorder' [8, 9]. This misconception is blurring the whole debate on diagnosis, classification, epidemiology, and treatment of PE. In 2006, Waldinger and Schweitzer emphasized the relevance of distinguishing between PE as a 'complaint' versus PE as a 'syndrome' [10–12]. PE as a 'complaint' may belong to the *normal* variation of ejaculatory performance in a certain number of men, but may also be the manifestation of medically or psychologically determined *pathological* ejaculatory performance. A 'syndrome' is defined as a cluster of symptoms and may give rise to a cluster of 'complaints'. For example, lifelong PE is a 'syndrome' as it gives rise to a cluster of various complaints that is similar in a large group of men. In contrast, there are also men who complain of PE but lack the whole symptomatology of men with lifelong PE. They report experiencing early ejaculations only occasionally. In other words, the latter men have 'complaints' of PE which are not part of an underlying syndrome or disorder. A nondistinction between complaint and disorder leads to misunderstanding of for example the epidemiology of PE [8, 9]. For example, it has become customary to start an article on PE with the following introduction: 'PE is the most prevalent male sexual *disorder* affecting some 20–30% of men'. This sentence mirrors a general belief that PE always represents a male sexual 'disorder'. However, if one distinguishes PE as a 'complaint' versus PE as a 'disorder', it appears more appropriate to state 'PE is the most prevalent male sexual *complaint* affecting some 20–30% of men. The prevalence of PE as a sexual *disorder* has not yet been investigated in the general male population, but is assumed to be much lower'.

What Is PE?

Theoretically, a man does not have PE when he has normal control over ejaculation. As he is able to control ejaculation, he is able to delay ejaculation until the moment he decides to ejaculate. In contrast, in case that control over ejaculation is insufficient, and a man can only ejaculate very shortly after penetration, it is generally agreed that he has PE. But oppositely, if a man has no control over ejaculation, and cannot delay ejaculation, but ejaculates a long time after penetration, this individual has no PE unless we define PE as a lack of control over ejaculation irrespectively whether ejaculation occurs shortly or long after penetration [13]. Therefore, agreement on 'what is PE', is dependent on how PE is defined. In short, PE can be defined in two different ways, namely, by 'objective criteria' and by 'subjective experiences'. A typical 'objective' criterion is the actual duration of the ejaculation time and the number of penile strokes. 'Subjective experiences', are for example a definition including any man who ejaculates before he or his partner 'wishes it', since he experienced 'diminished feelings of control' over his ejaculation, and/or this has caused him 'distress', 'dissatisfaction' or 'interpersonal difficulties'. These opposite paradigms have played a role in the development of the currently accepted DSM-IV-TR definition of PE.

DSM-III and DSM-IV-TR

In the DSM-III, published by the American Psychiatric Association in 1980, PE was defined as 'ejaculation that occurs before the individual wishes it, because of recurrent and persistent absence of reasonable *voluntary control* of ejaculation and orgasm during sexual activity'. However, due to disagreement on the criterion of 'reasonable voluntary control', this criterion was removed in the DSM-III-R in 1987 and later DSM-IV editions and replaced by the criterion of a 'short ejaculation time'. According to the DSM-IV-TR, published in 2000, PE is a 'persistent or recurrent ejaculation with minimal sexual stimulation before, on, or *shortly after* penetration and before the person wishes it. The clinician must take into account factors that affect duration of the excitement phase, such as age, novelty of the sexual partner or situation, and recent frequency of sexual activity' and requires for the diagnosis that 'the disturbance causes marked distress or interpersonal difficulty'. In other words, the DSM-III contains the criterion control and not the criterion of time. In contrast, the DSM-IV-TR contains the criterion of time and not the criterion of control. However, a cut-off point to quantify the 'short' ejaculation time has not been provided. In other words, the DSM-IV-TR attempts to be objective by using the criterion of a 'short' ejaculation time but also failed in it by not providing a cut-off point.

International Classification of Diseases (ICD-10)

The ICD-10, issued by the World Health Organization in 1992, defines PE as 'the inability to *control* ejaculation sufficiently for both partners to enjoy sexual interaction' and as 'an inability to *delay* ejaculation sufficiently to enjoy lovemaking, and manifest as either of the following: (1) occurrence of ejaculation before or *very soon after* the beginning of intercourse (if a time limit is required: before or within 15 s of the beginning of intercourse) and (2) ejaculation occurs in the absence of sufficient erection to make intercourse possible. In other words, the ICD-10 uses both the criterion of 'control' and the criterion of a 'very short' ejaculation time, and quantifies the ejaculation time to maximally 15 s after penetration. However, references to research supporting this quantification have not been provided. Interestingly, by using both criteria, the ICD-10 restricts the use of the criterion of control by the criterion of an ejaculation that occurs within 15 s. It should be noted that, by using the 15 s cut-off point, the ICD-10 provides an objective definition of PE.

What Is a 'Short' Ejaculation Time?

Both the DSM-IV-TR and the ICD-10 define PE in terms of a 'short' and even 'very short' ejaculation time after penetration. And although diminished feelings of control are not a criterion to diagnose PE according to the DSM-IV-TR, the ICD-10 uses the criterion of time to restrict the application of the criterion of control [13].

But what is a '(very) short' ejaculation time? In a clinical study in 110 men with lifelong PE [14], the duration of the ejaculation time was operationalized by the use of a stopwatch that was handled by the female partner; 90% of men ejaculated within 1 minute and 10% between 1 and 3 min. About 40% of men ejaculated within 15 s after penetration, which is the cut-off point of the ICD-10. As PE is not a life-threatening disorder, it was decided to set the cut-off point at 90%. Accordingly, the (very) short ejaculation time criterion was operationalized as being 1 min after penetration.

According to the participating couples, the use of a stopwatch did not interfere with sexual intercourse [14]. Recently, the 1 minute cut-off point was confirmed in another cohort of 88 men with lifelong PE who were actively seeking medical treatment and reported self-perceived ejaculation time [15].

However, in order to investigate whether the 1 min cut-off point is in the normal or abnormal range of the IELT of men in the general population, a stopwatch study in a random group of 491 men in 5 countries was conducted [16]. The study showed that the IELT in the general population had a positively skewed distribution with a median IELT of 5.4 min (range, 0.55–44.1 min) [16]. By using the 0.5 and 2.5 percentiles as statistical standards of what may be considered as normal or abnormal, it appeared that IELTs of less than 1 and 1.5 min are considered as abnormal in Western men [17]. This result confirms that men with IELTs of less than 1 min, indeed have abnormally short IELTs compared to men in the general population.

Risks of a Definition without an Operationalized IELT Cut-Off Point

Although it is clear that the DSM-IV-TR definition of PE requires a *short* ejaculation time, the absence of a cutoff point may lead to false-positive diagnoses of PE. For example, the existence of men who complain of PE while at the same time having normal and even long durations of the IELT became evident in two observational PE studies in the USA [18] and in Europe [19] in which clinicians diagnosed PE according to the DSM-IV-TR criteria of PE, added with questions about control and satisfaction, while ignoring the short ejaculation time criterion. As a result, in both studies about 45% of men had IELTs of 2–25 min when measured with a stopwatch. Obviously, it is very disputable to diagnose PE in men with normal (median IELT 5.4 min [16]) and long (5–25 min) IELT durations. As a result, these studies included a large number of men with false-positive diagnoses of PE. In recent years, it has become clear that the DSM-IV-TR definition of PE is inadequate and should be changed in the pending DSM-V [10, 11, 20–23].

Proposal for a New Classification of PE

Recently, a new proposal for the pending DSM-V and ICD-11 definition of PE has been put forward [8–13]. According to this proposal, PE should be classified according to a 'syndromal' approach incorporating well-controlled clinical and epidemiological stopwatch studies. PE as a clinical entity or a syndrome has for the first time been described by Bernhard Schapiro in 1943. He distinguished types A and B that were later termed 'lifelong' and 'acquired' PE by Godpodinoff. Both types have been mentioned but not further operationalized in the DSM-IV-TR definition of PE.

Recently, the existence of two other PE syndromes has been proposed, 'natural variable PE' [8–13] and 'premature-like ejaculatory dysfunction' [8–13]. In natural variable PE, men only occasionally suffer from early ejaculations. This should be regarded as part of the normal variability of ejaculatory performance and not a symptom of pathology. As such, natural variable PE is not a real syndrome. In premature-like ejaculatory dysfunction men experience and/or utter complaints of PE, while having objective normal or long durations of the IELT of 3–20 min. In the new proposal, the four PE syndromes are defined according to the following symptomatology.

Lifelong PE

Lifelong PE is a syndrome characterized by the cluster of the following core symptoms: (1) ejaculation occurs too early at nearly every intercourse, (2) with (nearly) every woman, (3) from about the first sexual encounters onwards, (4) in the majority of cases (90%) within 30–60 s, or between 1–2 min (10%) and remains rapid during life (70%) or can even aggravate during aging (30%) and, (3) the ability to delay ejaculation, i.e. to withhold ejaculation at the moment of imminent ejaculation may be diminished or lacking.

Some men already get an ejaculation during foreplay, before penetration (ejaculation ante portas), or soon as their penis touches the vagina (ejaculation intra portas). It should be noted that there are no hard indications that lifelong PE can be cured, neither by drug treatment or psychotherapy. In other words, lifelong PE is a chronic ejaculatory dysfunction. However, drug treatment may diminish the symptoms by the induced delayed ejaculation.

Acquired PE

The complaints of acquired PE differ in relation to the underlying somatic or psychological problem. It is characterized by the following symptoms. (1) early ejaculation occurs at some point in a man's life, (2) the man has usually had normal ejaculation experiences before the start of complaints, (3) there is either a sudden or gradual onset, (4) the ability to delay ejaculation, i.e. to withhold ejaculation at the moment of imminent ejaculation may be diminished or lacking, (5) the dysfunction may be due to urological dysfunctions like erectile dysfunction or prostatitis, thyroid dysfunction and psychological or relationship problems. In contrast to lifelong PE the acquired form of PE can be cured by treatment of the underlying cause.

Natural Variable PE

In natural variable PE, men only coincidentally and situationally experience early ejaculations. This type of PE should not be regarded as a symptom or manifestation of true pathology but of normal variation in sexual performance. The syndrome is characterized by the following symptoms. (1) early ejaculations are inconsistent and occur irregularly, (2) the ability to delay ejaculation, i.e. to withhold ejaculation at the moment of imminent ejaculation may be diminished or lacking, (3) experiences of diminished ability to delay ejaculation go along with either a short or normal ejaculation time, i.e an ejaculation of less or more than 1.5 min.

Premature-Like Ejaculatory Dysfunction

Men with premature-like ejaculatory dysfunction experience or complain of PE while the ejaculation time is in the normal range, i.e. around 3–6 min, and may even be of

	Lifelong PE	Acquired PE	Natural variable PE	Premature-like ejaculatory dysfunction
1	Very short IELT	(Very) short IELT	Normal IELT	Normal/long IELT
2	Neurobiological genetic	Medical psychological	Normal variation	Psychological
3	Medication	Medication psychotherapy	Reassurance	Psychotherapy
4	Low prevalence	Low prevalence	High prevalence	High prevalence

Fig. 1. Continuum of the four PE syndromes. Lifelong PE is more neurobiologically determined while premature-like ejaculatory dysfunction is more psychologically determined. 1 = Duration IELT, 2 = etiology, 3 = treatment, 4 = prevalence.

very long duration, i.e. between 5–25 min. This type of PE should not be regarded as a symptom or manifestation of true medical pathology. Psychological and/or relationship problems may underlie the complaints. The syndrome is characterized by the following symptoms.

(1) Subjective perception of consistent or inconsistent rapid ejaculation during intercourse. (2) Preoccupation with an imagined early ejaculation or lack of control of ejaculation. (3) The actual IELT is in the normal range or may even be of longer duration (i.e. an ejaculation that occurs between 5 and 25 min). (4) The ability to delay ejaculation, i.e. to withhold ejaculation at the moment of imminent ejaculation may be diminished or lacking. (5) The preoccupation is not better accounted for by another mental disorder.

Continuum of Neurobiology and Psychology

The distinction of the four PE syndromes shows a continuum of PE along a line from mainly neurobiologically to mainly psychologically determined forms (fig. 1). For example, from both human and animal research it may be derived that lifelong PE is presumably highly neurobiologically and perhaps also genetically determined. However, as yet one cannot rule out that certain forms of lifelong PE are psychologically determined. Like is the case in major depression, a biological marker of lifelong PE has not yet been found. However, the positive response on daily SSRI drug treatment indicates that both major depression and PE are neurobiologically, i.e. serotonergically, mediated and may have a neurobiological etiology. Acquired PE may be medically (prostatitis, thyroid dysfunction) or psychologically (relationship problems) determined. The sporadic early ejaculations in natural variable PE have been postulated to represent the normal variation of ejaculatory performance in men and are presumably not an expression of underlying pathology. The complaints of early ejaculations in men with premature-like ejaculatory dysfunction which occur at normal and even long durations of the IELT, have been postulated to be due to mainly psychological factors.

Prevalence of PE

Epidemiological research has repeatedly shown a prevalence of PE of 20–30% [24]. Erroneously, by not distinguishing PE as a complaint and as a syndrome, it has been concluded that the 'disorder' PE has a high prevalence. However, these studies have only shown that the 'complaint' of PE in the general male population has a high prevalence of 20–30%. Studies into the prevalence of lifelong PE and acquired PE have never been conducted. However, it is of note that the prevalence of lifelong PE, defined in terms of lifelong consistent IELTs of less than 1–1.5 min along feelings of diminished ability to delay ejaculation, has been suggested to be rather low (2–5%). Further epidemiological research to confirm this hypothesis is warranted. It is suggested that in case the prevalence of lifelong PE appears to be rather low, it should be argued that only a small percentage of men with 'complaints' of PE suffer from PE that is mainly neurobiologically and genetically determined [8, 9]. This is of major importance for genetic studies on PE. New epidemiological research may also contribute to confirm the hypothesis that the high percentage of 'complaints' of PE (20–30%) is due to the large number of males in the general population that either have natural variable PE or premature-like ejaculatory dysfunction.

Pathophysiology of PE

The distinction of the four PE syndromes illustrates that there is not one particular pathophysiology of PE, but that there are different pathophysiologies dependent on the type of PE [13, 14]. For example, the serotonin hypothesis of PE, i.e. a disturbance of serotonin neurotransmission and/or serotonin receptor functioning [1], pertains only to lifelong PE and partly to acquired PE, as the persistently and objectively very short ejaculation time is likely to be the symptom of a neurobiological dysfunction. In other words, the serotonin hypothesis explains probably only a small percentage (2–5%) of complaints of PE in the general population. The pathophysiology of acquired PE is related to disturbances of peripheral neuronal functioning, whereas the pathophysiology of premature-like ejaculatory dysfunction is speculated to be related to cognitive and unconscious mental process disturbances and not the result of a biological disturbance as the ejaculation time is normal.

Diagnosis of the PE Syndromes

Lifelong, acquired, natural variable PE and premature-like ejaculatory dysfunction are recognizable by taking a brief medical and sexual history with special attention to the duration of the ejaculation time, the frequency of occurrences and the course since the first sexual encounters. In daily clinical practice, diagnosis of the four PE syndromes is not difficult and therefore evaluation with questionnaires or the use of a stopwatch is not required. However, for drug treatment trials and epidemiological research, stopwatch assessment and questionnaires of satisfaction and quality of (sexual) life are a prerequisite.

New Definition of PE

The distinction of the four PE syndromes is important for a new classification of PE. As the four syndromes differ in symptomatology, each of these syndromes should be separately defined. Of the four syndromes, most evidence-based research on PE has been conducted on men with lifelong PE. In October 2007, a new definition on lifelong PE has been formulated and accepted with general approval at a consensus meeting of the International Society of Sexual Medicine in Amsterdam. According to this new definition, PE is a male sexual dysfunction characterized by ejaculation, which always or nearly always occurs prior to or within about 1 min of vaginal penetration, and the inability to delay ejaculation on all or nearly all vaginal penetrations, and, which has negative personal consequences, such as distress, bother, frustration and/or the avoidance of sexual intimacy.

Neurobiology

The very strong ejaculation-delaying effects of daily SSRI treatment has contributed to a better understanding of the involvement of the central serotonergic system in the SSRI-induced ejaculation delay. However, although the serotonergic system and other neurotransmitter systems, like the dopaminergic and oxytocinergic systems, are involved in drug-induced delay of ejaculation, and it is assumed that these central neurotransmitter systems also play a role in the pathophysiology of PE, the neurobiology of PE is still unknown. For a better understanding of the strong ejaculation-delaying effects of daily SSRI treatment and the minimal ejaculation-delaying effects of on-demand SSRI treatment, some basic knowledge of central serotonergic metabolism is pivotal.

Serotonin Neurotransmission and Serotonergic Receptors

Serotonergic (5-hydroxytryptamine; 5-HT) neurons regulate their own activity by three mechanisms [25]. Under normal physiological conditions, endogenous somatodendritic release of 5-HT activates (presynaptic) 5-HT_{1A} autoreceptors that are present on the cell bodies and dendrites of serotonergic neurons in the raphe nuclei of the brainstem (fig. 2). Activation of these 5-HT_{1A} autoreceptors decreases firing of the 5-HT neuron and consequently lowers the 5-HT release from the presynaptic neuron into the synaptic cleft (mechanism 1). After release of 5-HT in the synapse, presynaptic 5-HT_{1B} autoreceptors become activated, which in turn inhibits the 5-HT release

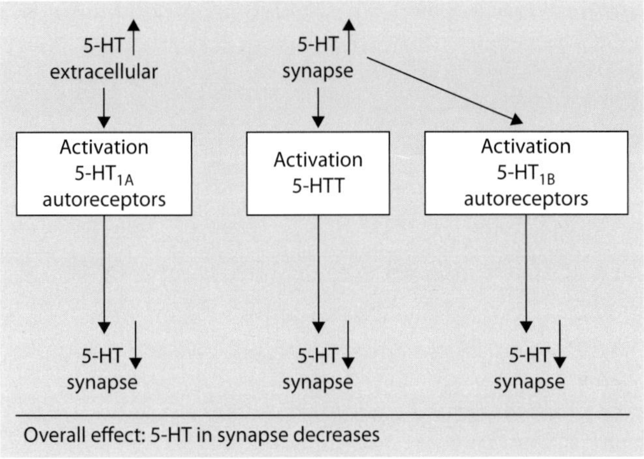

Fig. 2. Three automechanisms of the serotonergic neuron to prevent overstimulation of postsynaptic 5-HT receptors when 5-HT increases in the synapse and extracellularly.

from the presynaptic neuron into the synaptic cleft (mechanism 2). This feedback mechanism of the neuron probably prevents overstimulation of (post)synaptic 5-HT receptors. Another automechanism to prevent overstimulation of postsynaptic 5 HT receptors is the immediate removal of 5-HT in the synapse back into the presynaptic neuron by 5-HT transporters (5-HTTs), which are not only present at the presynaptic endings but also at the serotonergic cell bodies and dendrites (mechanism 3).

Acute and Chronic Administration of SSRIs

Acute Administration. All 5-HT transporters are blocked after acute SSRI administration leading to higher 5-HT levels in the synaptic cleft and in the extracellular space around the cell bodies of 5-HT-containing nerves. The increased extracellular 5-HT levels activate 5-HT_{1A} autoreceptors and consequently lead to lower 5-HT release into the synaptic cleft within minutes. The diminished release of 5-HT in the synaptic cleft compensates (completely or partially) the initially increased 5-HT concentrations as the result of the SSRI-induced blockade of the 5-HT reuptake by transporters from the synaptic cleft into the presynaptic neuron. Higher 5-HT concentrations in the synapse will increase the activation of presynaptic 5-HT_{1B} autoreceptors that by itself will attenuate 5-HT release. The net effect of acute SSRI administration, under physiological conditions, is only a mild or no increase of 5-HT neurotransmission and mild or no stimulation of all postsynaptic 5-HT receptors (fig. 3).

Chronic Administration. Chronic administration of SSRIs leads to a number of adaptations. The ongoing blockade of 5-HTTs results in a persistent increase of 5-HT levels in the synaptic cleft and around somatodendritic cell bodies. This leads to

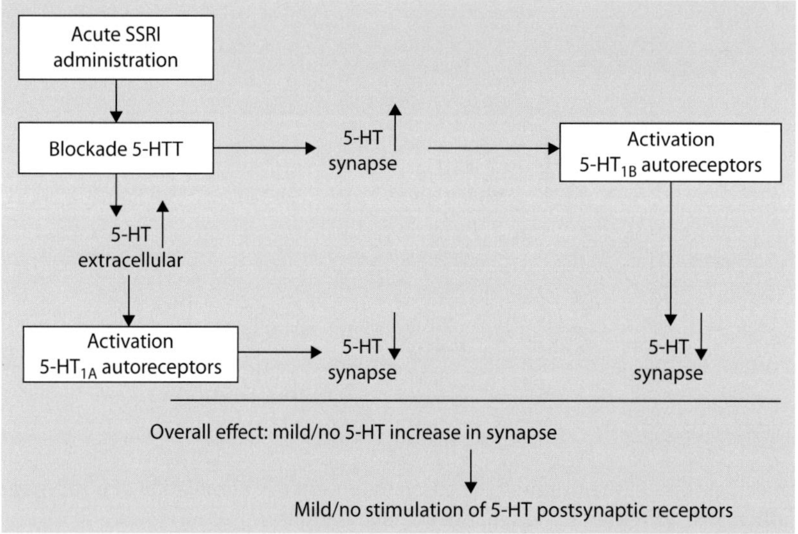

Fig. 3. Acute SSRI administration leads to mild or even no increased 5-HT neurotransmission and to mild or even no stimulation of postsynaptic 5-HT receptors.

desensitization of 5-HT_{1A} autoreceptors over the course of 2 weeks, possibly also desensitization of 5-HT_{1B} autoreceptors, and consequently to less inhibition of 5-HT release into the synaptic cleft. The net effect of chronic SSRI administration is thus a stronger enhancement of 5-HT neurotransmission with a consequently stronger activation of postsynaptic 5-HT receptors compared with acute SSRI administration (fig. 4).

Serotonergic, Dopaminergic and Oxytocinergic System

Various neurotransmitters, like serotonin, dopamine, and oxytocine are involved in the ejaculatory process [26]. It might well be that these three neurotransmitter systems are also involved in the pathophysiology of PE at least when PE is defined in terms of a persistently very short (i.e. less than 1 min) ejaculation time concurrent with a persistent inability to delay ejaculation. Only in these men is it assumed that a neurobiological dysfunction underlies the very short IELT.

Evidence-Based Research

In the last decade, an evidence-based drug treatment methodology and statistics have been developed by independent researchers. Apart from randomized, double-blind placebo-controlled study designs, drug treatment studies of PE should include a baseline and a drug treatment period in which the IELT is measured prospectively at each coitus using a stopwatch handled by the female partner. Drug-induced adverse effects should be assessed with a validated questionnaire. Moreover, side effects of on-demand

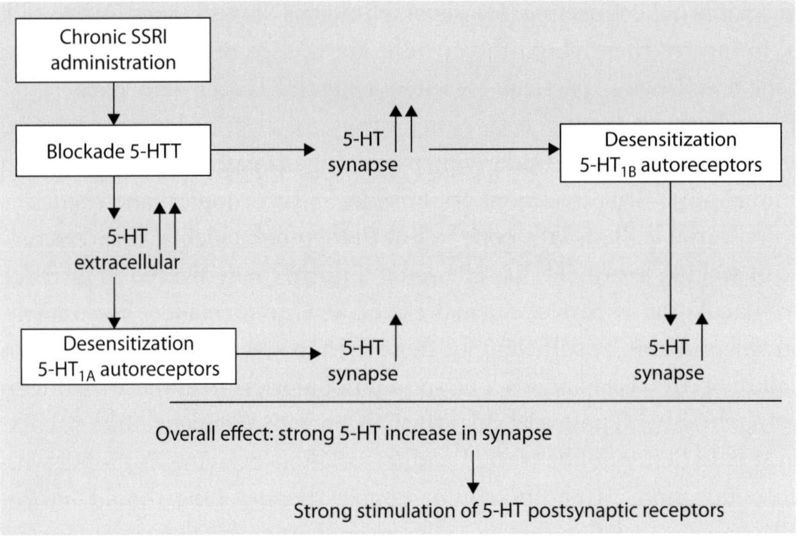

Fig. 4. Chronic SSRI administration leads to strong increased 5-HT neurotransmission and strong stimulation of postsynaptic 5-HT receptors.

treatment should be assessed at the day of drug intake and the next day, i.e. within 24–48 h after drug intake.

Because ejaculation-delaying drugs give rise to positive skewness of the IELT distribution, the IELT values should be logarithmically transformed and results should be reported as geometric mean IELT or median IELT. In addition, ejaculation delay should be expressed as percentage or fold increase from baseline with 95% confidence intervals. It is of note that placebo and very weak ejaculation-delaying drugs may give rise to a normal IELT distribution or a very weak skewed IELT distribution. In this case, the values of the mean IELT, median IELT and geometric mean IELT hardly differ from each other. In contrast, in moderate and strong ejaculation-delaying drugs these values differ from each other, whereby the geometric mean IELT < median IELT < mean IELT. The stronger the drug delays ejaculation, the higher the differences between these values. In other words, ejaculation delay in those cases should not be expressed by the mean IELT as this overestimates the real ejaculation delay which should be expressed by the geometric mean IELT [27].

Treatment

The distinction of the four PE syndromes has consequences for treatment. Lifelong PE should be treated with drugs that strongly delay ejaculation. It is a matter of debate whether additional counseling is always needed for these men. A lot of these men will manage without additional counseling. However, clinicians should take time to talk with these men, to inform them about the current knowledge of lifelong PE and to regularly check their well-being, particularly when using SSRIs on a daily basis.

Acquired PE needs to be treated with either drugs to treat underlying medical pathology, or psychotherapy to treat underlying psychological pathology, or both with or without additional other drug treatment options like SSRIs or topical anesthetics.

Men with natural variable PE usually cope well with their coincidental early ejaculations, but in case of seeking treatment, it is advised to inform them that the occurrence of sporadic early ejaculation is part of normal ejaculatory performance. Presumably, psychoeducation will probably be sufficient for these men to regain confidence. Due to the incidental nature of early ejaculations, one should not a priori treat these men with ejaculation-delaying drugs with potential side effects. Men with Premature-like ejaculatory dysfunction should better not be treated with ejaculation-delaying drugs but with counseling, psychoeducation, psychotherapy or couple therapy. One should inform these men that the actual ejaculation time is in the normal range but that psychological or relationship factors are likely to contribute to their complaint.

Daily SSRI Treatment

During the last decade, daily use of SSRIs, on-demand use of the tricyclic antidepressant clomipramine and topical use of anesthetics has become most popular to treat PE [28]. Although none of these treatment options have been approved by the Food and Drug Administration, their use has been recognized and is supported by evidence-based studies [28]. The serotonergic antidepressants modify the course of PE by modulating the central serotonergic system and the anesthetics suppress the sensitivity of the glans penis. A number of studies further reported efficacy of the on-demand use of phosphodiesterase type 5 (PDE-5) inhibitors but their role in the treatment of PE without erectile dysfunction is disputable. Recently, two studies reported ejaculation-delaying effects of the on-demand use of tramadol. Actually, one can distinguish two major strategies to treat PE by medication; daily and on-demand treatment.

Daily Treatment with Clomipramine

In 1973, Eaton published the first publication on the efficacy of clomipramine, the most serotonergic tricyclic antidepressant, to treat PE. Particularly, in the 1970–1980s but also in the 1990s various studies demonstrated its efficacy in delaying ejaculation in rather low daily dosages of 10–30 mg.

Daily Treatment with SSRIs

The introduction of the SSRIs in psychiatry however, would lead to a revolutionary chance in the understanding of and treatment of PE. After the first publication in 1994 [4] on the efficacy of daily treatment with paroxetine hemihydrate, various studies confirmed its strong ejaculation-delaying effects at dosages of 20–40 mg [29].

Moreover, it appeared that nearly all SSRIs, except fluvoxamine, exerted a clinically relevant ejaculation delaying effect [28]. Currently, daily treatment with SSRIs or combined daily treatment with on-demand use of some SSRIs has become the first choice of treatment. In 2004, Waldinger et al. [28] published a systematic review and meta-analysis of all drug treatment studies that have been published between 1943 and 2003. Of all 79 studies, a meta-analysis was only feasible on 35 clomipramine and SSRI daily treatment studies that were conducted between 1973 and 2003 [28]. The outcome data of the few SSRI treatment studies published between 2003 and 2007 hardly distort the findings of the systematic review and meta-analysis, and therefore its conclusions are still valid today. The meta-analysis revealed a placebo effect of a geometric mean 1.4-fold IELT increase (95% CI: 1.2–1.7). Furthermore, it was demonstrated that the rank order of efficacy (geometric mean fold increase of IELT) was (a) paroxetine (8.8; 95% CI: 5.9–13.2), (b) clomipramine (4.6; 3.0–7.4), (c) sertraline (4.1; 2.6–7.0) and (d) fluoxetine (3.9; 3.0–5.4). Thus, in general, daily SSRI treatment studies generate a 2.6- to 13.2-fold increase in geometric mean IELT, depending on the type of SSRI. Daily treatment can be performed with paroxetine 20–40 mg, clomipramine 10–50 mg, sertraline 50–100 mg, fluoxetine 20–40 mg, citalopram 20–40 mg and 10–20 mg escitalopram. Ejaculation delay usually starts a few days after drug intake, but becomes more manifest after 1–2 weeks. The delay continues to exist for years, but sometimes may diminish after 6–12 months. The cause of this tachyphylaxis of SSRIs has not yet been clarified [29].

Daily SSRI treatment is most often, but not always, effective in delaying ejaculation. The reason that SSRIs sometimes fail to delay ejaculation has not yet been clarified. Patients should be informed about the short-term and long-term side effects of SSRIs. In the short-term, fatigue, yawning, mild nausea, loose stools or perspiration may occur. These side effects are usually mild, start in the first 1–2 weeks of treatment, and most often gradually disappear within 2–3 weeks. Although a head-to-head comparative study has not yet been performed, drug treatment studies seem to indicate that in contrast to the side effects in depressed patients, diminished libido and erectile dysfunction are less frequently and also to a lesser extent reported by healthy non-depressed men with lifelong PE. A rather rare side effect of SSRIs is the risk of bleeding. Clinicians should warn patients about combining SSRIs with aspirin or NSAIDs as this may further increase the risk of bleeding. A very rare side effect is priapism. Although very rare, it is advised to inform all patients using SSRIs about the risk of priapism and its need for immediate medical treatment. One should not prescribe these drugs to young men < 18 years, and to men known with depressive disorder particularly when associated with suicidal thoughts. In those cases, referral to a psychiatrist is indicated. In the long-term, weight gain might occur with an associated risk for diabetes mellitus type II.

Patients should be advised not to stop taking the medication acutely to prevent the occurrence of an SSRI discontinuation syndrome, which is characterized by symptoms like tremor, shock-like sensations when turning the head, nausea and dizziness.

Generic versus Brand-Name SSRIs

A special note should be made to the use of generic SSRIs. The most relevant studies on SSRI treatment of PE have been conducted in the early and mid-90s using the brand-name SSRIs, simply because at that time generic SSRIs were not yet on the market. In contrast, today generic SSRIs are frequently prescribed. In a review of the few publications comparing the bioequivalence and efficacy of brand-name and generic psychoactive drugs, it was shown that there are differences between the generic drugs and the brand-name drugs which had not been noted in the original bioequivalence studies. This issue has consequences for drug treatment of PE.

Paroxetine Hemihydrate

Daily treatment of PE with paroxetine has been investigated with paroxetine hydrochloride hemihydrate and not with the generic drug paroxetine hemihydrate and/or paroxetine mesylate. The ejaculation-delaying efficacy and relatively mild side effect profile of paroxetine hemihydrate have been repeatedly demonstrated in well-controlled studies. Based on these studies, there are no real objective contraindications to use the generic paroxetine hemihydrate to treat PE.

Paroxetine Mesylate

Drug treatment studies on PE have not been performed with paroxetine *mesylate*. There are some indications that particularly the side-effect profile of the generic paroxetine-mesylate is different from paroxetine hemihydrates. Therefore, and due to the lack of placebo-controlled comparative studies investigating the efficacy and side effect profile of both paroxetine hemihydrate and paroxetine mesylate in the treatment of PE, it is advised to prescribe only paroxetine hydrochloride hemihydrate to men with lifelong PE and not paroxetine mesylate.

Daily Treatment with α_1-Adrenoceptor Antagonists

Ejaculation is peripherally controlled by the sympathetic nervous system. Blocking the sympathetic system by α_1-adrenoceptor antagonists (α_1-blockers) may theoretically delay ejaculation. Terazosin and alfuzosin are two selective α_1-blockers whose ejaculation-delaying effects have been investigated in men with PE. In a placebo-controlled study in 91 men with PE, both terazosin 5 mg/day and alfuzosin 6 mg/day proved effective in approximately 50% of the cases. In another placebo-controlled study in 90 men with PE and lower urinary tract symptoms without chronic prostatitis and benign prostatic hyperplasia, daily use of terazosin 5–10 mg showed a clinically significant improvement. However, the methodology of both studies has been rather weak. Efficacy was measured by merely qualitative measures like satisfaction and subjective feelings of improvement. Prolongation of the IELT was not assessed by a stopwatch. Although α_1-blockers may affect ejaculatory performance, they do not always delay ejaculation. Despite the aforementioned limitations in methodology and the rather low rate of clinically relevant ejaculation-delaying effects, α_1-blockers, and particularly terazosin 5–10 mg may be a good alternative to treat men with PE who also have urinary tract dysfunction. However, further well-designed studies are pivotal to evaluate the place of α_1-blockers in the armentarium of drugs in the treatment of PE.

On-Demand Drug Treatment

Despite any study investigating patient preferences, it has recently become rather fashionable to state that on-demand treatment of PE would be more favorable than daily treatment. This is rather peculiar as contrary to daily treatment, on-demand strategies may quite negatively interfere with the spontaneity of having sex, particularly as one usually decides to have sex at the spur of the moment. This is particularly so in young adults with children when the couple often take the opportunity to have sex at a sudden moment when the chance to be disturbed is very low. Also the argument that daily treatment is not preferable because one has to wait 1–2 weeks before ejaculation delay occurs is not based on evidence. Most men with lifelong PE will report that after many years of having had PE, it is no problem to wait another 1–2 weeks before medication becomes effective. Moreover, a clear advantage of daily treatment is that ejaculation is delayed at every moment of the day that one wished to have intercourse. Recently, the first study was published investigating the preferences of men with lifelong PE for the currently existing PE treatment options [15]. In this study in 88 men with lifelong PE, it was shown that 81% preferred *daily* drug treatment mainly because patients feared that on-demand treatment would negatively interfere with the spontaneity of having sex [15].

Nevertheless, on-demand drug treatment contributes to the armentarium of drug treatment of PE. In recent years, on-demand treatment studies have been conducted with topical anesthetics, clomipramine, SSRIs, dapoxetine, tramadol, and PDE-5 inhibitors. Due to differences in methodology and design, a meta-analysis comparing the efficacy of these drugs has not yet been feasible.

On-Demand Treatment with Topical Anesthetics

The use of topical local anesthetics such as lidocaine and/or prilocaine in the form of a cream, gel or spray is the oldest drug treatment strategy and is still practiced today. The topical anesthetics delay ejaculation by reducing the sensitivity of the glans penis. However, only a few studies have been conducted to show their efficacy. The application is rather simple, but still may lead to side effects like complete anesthesia of the penis which may lead to erectile difficulties. Patients should be informed that its use may also lead to vaginal numbness. This may be prevented by the use of a condom.

On-Demand Treatment with Clomipramine

On-demand use of 20–40 mg clomipramine can effectively delay ejaculation after 3–5 h. However, it might also give rise to nausea at the day of intercourse and the next day.

On-Demand Treatment with SSRIs

In the systematic review of 2003, only eight studies on on-demand treatment with SSRIs and clomipramine were reported [28]. These eight on-demand studies greatly differed in methodology. A meta-analysis on the published on-demand SSRI studies could not be performed as the studies were unbalanced for the antidepressants used, baseline IELT values, design (double-blind versus open) and assessment techniques (questionnaire versus stopwatch) [28]. In spite of the absence of a meta-analysis on on-demand SSRI treatment studies, there are indications that on-demand use of SSRIs, like 20 mg paroxetine, do not strongly delay ejaculation after 3–5 h of intake [28].

On-Demand Treatment with Dapoxetine

Recently, a multicenter study with dapoxetine, an SSRI with a short half-life, has shown that despite minimal ejaculation delay, objectivated with stopwatch assessment, feelings of satisfaction and control were improved [30]. However, the methodology of investigating side effects in this study and the statistics that were used to describe ejaculation delay have given rise to a debate in sexual medicine literature. The side effects were retrospectively reported at each monthly visit to the clinic. A better methodology would have been a prospective assessment within 24–48 h after drug intake. The dapoxetine-induced ejaculation delay was expressed as mean IELT, suggesting a normal IELT distribution. As investigations with placebo and conventional SSRIs have suggested that normal or very weak skewed IELT distribution indicate a very weak ejaculation-delaying effect, it may be derived that dapoxetine has a very weak ejaculation-delaying effect [6, 7, 27, 31].

On-Demand Treatment with Tramadol

Recently, two studies in men with PE have shown the ejaculation-delaying effects of on-demand use of 50 mg tramadol. Tramadol is registered as a centrally acting analgesic agent combining μ-opioid receptor activation and reuptake inhibition of serotonin and noradrenaline. The most common adverse effects of tramadol were nausea (15.6%), vomiting (6.2%) and dizziness (6.2%), but they were reported to be mild. However, it should be noted that although tramadol has a weak μ-opioid agonistic effect, long-term follow-up studies are also needed to investigate the risk of opioid addiction.

On-Demand Treatment with PDE-5 Inhibitors

In recent years, a number of authors have suggested that on-demand use of PDE-5 inhibitors is effective in treating PE. However, most of these studies lack a good methodology which makes the results difficult to interpret. Recently, McMahon et al. [32] published a well-designed systematic review of all publications on the use of PDE-5 inhibitors against PE that have been published between 2001 until 2006. The review analyzed 14 studies, which reported the use of sildenafil, vardenafil, and tadalafil. The majority of these studies did not fulfill the current criteria of evidence-based medicine. Of the 14 studies, only one fulfilled these criteria. It was concluded that there is no convincing evidence of any direct effect of PDE-5 inhibitors on the central or peripheral control of ejaculation, or for any role in the treatment of PE, except for men with PE and comorbid erectile dysfunction [32].

On-Demand Treatment with Intracavernous Vasoactive Drug Injection
A special comment should be made regarding intracavernous self-injection treatment. This strategy to treat PE is advocated by a few institutions. However, it should be noted that there is not any evidence-based support for the efficacy of this strategy. Actually, there has only been one single study investigating this treatment method. In this open study of 8 men, patients injected vasoactive drugs into the corpus cavernosum. From the 8 men, 3 stated that they were cured and stopped the treatment while the other 5 men continued using the medication after 14 months. However, the methodology of this study was very weak. There were no baseline assessments of the IELT, and a prolongation of the IELT was not measured with a stopwatch. Moreover, success of treatment was defined by prolongation of erectile function after ejaculation and not by the measure of a delayed ejaculation. As long as there are no well-controlled studies showing the efficacy of injection treatment to delay ejaculation time, one should not treat PE with intracavernosal injection of vasoactive drugs.

Conclusions

The lack of an evidence-based cut-off point of the short-ejaculation time criterion of the DSM-IV-TR definition of PE may form a risk for false-positive diagnoses of PE. Recently, a '1 min' criterion of a PE definition has gained general approval at a consensus meeting of the International Society of Sexual Medicine held in October 2007 in Amsterdam, but this criterion was restricted to lifelong PE. For the pending DSM-V a new classification of four PE syndromes has been proposed. According to this classification, PE can no longer be defined in one overall descriptive definition, but should be defined according to the symptomatology of the underlying PE syndrome.

The high prevalence rate of 20–30% is more likely to reflect the percentage of men that have 'complaints' of PE, rather than the percentage of men that suffer from the 'disorder' lifelong PE and acquired PE. The percentage of men that are in need for drug treatment is probably much lower than the high percentage of men than have 'complaints' of PE without suffering from PE syndromes. Similarly, it is likely that PE is neurobiologically and/or genetically determined only in a small percentage of cases. It has been suggested that a much higher percentage of men only occasionally experience early ejaculations, representing the normal variation of ejaculatory performance. Similarly, it has been suggested that presumably a high percentage of men complain of early ejaculation while having normal and even long durations of the

IELT. Treatment of PE is dependent of its etiology. Drug treatment is particularly indicated for men with lifelong PE and acquired PE. This may be combined with counseling or behavioral therapy. Psychotherapy is particularly indicated for men with premature-like ejaculatory dysfunction or secondary PE due to psychological problems. Psychoeducation should be provided to men with natural variable PE. Of the various drug treatment options, daily drug treatment with SSRIs, particularly paroxetine, on-demand use of clomipramine and/or topical anesthetics has become most popular and their efficacy has been based on evidence-based research.

References

1 Waldinger MD: The neurobiological approach to premature ejaculation. J Urol 2002;168:2359–2367.
2 Waldinger MD: Lifelong premature ejaculation: from authority-based to evidence-based medicine. Brit J Urol Int 2004;93:201–207.
3 Masters WH, Johnson VE: Premature ejaculation; in Masters WH, Johnson VE (eds): Human Sexual Inadequacy. Little, Brown, Boston 1970, pp 92–115.
4 Waldinger MD, Hengeveld MW, Zwinderman AH: Paroxetine treatment of premature ejaculation: a double-blind, randomized, placebo-controlled study. Am J Psychiatry 1994;151:1377–1379.
5 Waldinger MD: Towards evidence-based drug treatment research on premature ejaculation: a critical evaluation of methodology. J Impot Res 2003;15: 309–313.
6 Waldinger MD, Schweitzer DH: Premature ejaculation and pharmaceutical company-based medicine: the dapoxetine case. J Sex Med 2008; in press.
7 Waldinger MD, Schweitzer DH: Is Dapoxetine effective enough in delaying ejaculation in men with lifelong premature ejaculation? A critical review on the role of pharmaceutical companies. ISDB Newsletter 2008; in press.
8 Waldinger MD: Premature ejaculation: State of the art. Urol Clin North Am 2007;34:591–599.
9 Waldinger MD: Premature ejaculation: different pathophysiologies and etiologies determine its treatment. J Sex Marital Ther 2008;34:1–13.
10 Waldinger MD, Schweitzer DH: Changing paradigms from an historical DSM-III and DSM-IV view towards an evidence based definition of premature ejaculation. Part I: Validity of DSM-IV-TR. J Sex Med 2006;3:682–692.
11 Waldinger MD, Schweitzer DH: Changing paradigms from an historical DSM-III and DSM-IV view towards an evidence based definition of premature ejaculation. Part II: Proposals for DSM-V and ICD-11. J Sex Med 2006;3:693–705.
12 Waldinger MD: The need for a revival of psychoanalytic investigations into premature ejaculation. J Mens Health Gend 2006;3:390–396.
13 Waldinger MD, Schweitzer DH: The use of old and recent DSM definitions of premature ejaculation in observational studies: a contribution to the present debate for a new classification of PE in the DSM-V. J Sex Med 2008; in press.
14 Waldinger MD, Hengeveld MW, Zwinderman AH, Olivier B: An empirical operationalization study of DSM-IV diagnostic criteria for premature ejaculation. Intern J Psychiatry Clin Pract 1998;2:287–293.
15 Waldinger MD, Zwinderman AH, Olivier B, Schweitzer DH: The majority of men with lifelong premature ejaculation prefer daily drug treatment: an observational study in a consecutive group of Dutch men. J Sex Med 2007;4:1028–1037.
16 Waldinger MD, Quinn P, Dilleen M, Mundayat R, Schweitzer DH, Boolell M: A multinational population survey of intravaginal ejaculation latency time. J Sex Med 2005;2:492–497.
17 Waldinger MD, Zwinderman AH, Olivier B, Schweitzer DH: Proposal for a definition of lifelong premature ejaculation based on epidemiological stopwatch data. J Sex Med 2005;2:498–507.
18 Patrick DL, Althof SE, Pryor JL, Rosen R, Rowland DL, Ho KF, McNulty P, Rothman M, Jamieson C: Premature ejaculation: An observational study of men and their partners. J Sex Med 2005;2:358–367.
19 Giuliano F, Patrick DL, Porst H, La Pera G, Kokoszka A, Merchant S, Rothman M, Gagnon DD, Polverejan E for the 3004 Study Group: Premature ejaculation: results from a five-country European observational study. Eur Urol 2007; epub.
20 Waldinger MD, Schweitzer DH: The DSM-IV-TR is an inadequate diagnostic tool for premature ejaculation (letter). J Sex Med 2007;4:822–823.

21 Balon R, Segraves RT, Clayton A: Issues for DSM-V: Sexual dysfunction, disorder, or variation along normal distribution: Toward rethinking DSM criteria of sexual dysfunctions. Am J Psychiatry 2007; 164:198–199.

22 Segraves R, Balon R, Clayton A: Proposal for changes in diagnostic criteria for sexual dysfunctions. J Sex Med 2007;4:567–580.

23 Segraves RT, Balon R: Toward an improved nosology of sexual dysfunctions in DSM-V. Psychiatric Times 2007;24:44–46.

24 St. Lawrence JS, Madakasira S: Evaluation and treatment of premature ejaculation: a critical review. Int J Psychiatr Med 1992;22:77–97.

25 Olivier B, van Oorschot R, Waldinger MD: Serotonin, serotonergic receptors, selective serotonin reuptake inhibitors and sexual behaviour. Int Clin Psychopharmacol 1998;13 (suppl 6): S9–S14.

26 de Jong TR, Veening JG, Olivier B, Waldinger MD: Oxytocin involvement in SSRI-induced delayed ejaculation: a review of animal studies. J Sex Med 2007;4:14–28.

27 Waldinger MD, Zwinderman AH, Olivier B, Schweitzer DH: Geometric mean IELT and premature ejaculation: Appropriate statistics to avoid overestimation of treatment efficacy. J Sex Med 2008;5: 492–499.

28 Waldinger MD, Zwinderman AH, Schweitzer DH, Olivier B: Relevance of methodological design for the interpretation of efficacy of drug treatment of premature ejaculation: a systematic review and meta-analysis. Int J Impot Res 2004;16:369–381.

29 Waldinger MD: Premature ejaculation: definition and drug treatment. Drugs 2007;67:547–568.

30 Pryor JL, Althof SE, Steidle C, Rosen RC, Hellstrom WJG, Shabsigh R, Miloslavsky M, Kell S: Efficacy and tolerability of dapoxetine in treatment of premature ejaculation: an integrated analysis of two double-blind, randomised controlled trials. Lancet 2006;368:929–937.

31 Waldinger MD, Schweitzer DH, Olivier B: Dapoxetine treatment of premature ejaculation (Letter). Lancet 2006;368:1869–1870.

32 McMahon CG, McMahon CN, Liang JL, Winestock CG: Efficacy of type-5 phophodiesterase inhibitors in the drug treatment of premature ejaculation: a systematic review. BJU Int 2006;98:259–272.

Marcel D. Waldinger, MD, PhD
Department of Psychiatry and Neurosexology, HagaHospital Leyenburg
Leyweg 275
NL–2545 CH The Hague (The Netherlands)
Tel. +31 70 210 2086, Fax +31 70 210 4902, E-Mail md@waldinger.demon.nl

Balon R (ed): Sexual Dysfunction. The Brain-Body Connection.
Adv Psychosom Med. Basel, Karger, 2008, vol 29, pp 70–88

The Impact of Physical Illness on Sexual Dysfunction

Anita Clayton · Sujatha Ramamurthy

Department of Psychiatry and Neurobehavioral Sciences, University of Virginia, Charlottesville, Va., USA

Abstract

Sexuality is the ultimate union of mind and body. Sexual dysfunction is often the first manifestation of physical illness but is often not inquired about on routine review of symptoms. This is, in large part, due to the health care providers' lack of knowledge in diagnosis and treatment of sexual impairment as well as their discomfort with this sensitive topic. However, sexual well-being is an important determinant of quality of life and many medically ill patients find sexual intimacy to be an essential mode of communication with their partners. This chapter attempts to methodically delineate physical illnesses causing sexual dysfunction by organ system. Neurologic, endocrinologic, cardiovascular and pelvic illnesses are discussed as to their impact on sexual health. Diagnostic and established treatment strategies are also reviewed. Breast cancer, rheumatoid arthritis and psoriasis are touched upon. Although not a disease, pregnancy and its unique impact on sexuality is also discussed. Not only the disease itself but the treatment prescribed may also cause sexual impairment. Thus, a separate section on medications that impair sexual functioning is presented. A table of common medications as a quick reference to their effects on each stage of the sexual cycle is also provided.

Sexuality is the ultimate union of mind and body. Not surprisingly, illness in either realm often first manifests as sexual impairment. Only recently has modern medicine acknowledged the inseparable relationship between body and mind, and formal scientific inquiry has lagged behind. Thus, many diseases are fully described as to the effects on the specific organ systems involved, but not on how they influence sexuality. Also studying sexuality challenges the scientist to bring the most private, intimate interaction between people into the public, sterile laboratory environment in hopes of quantifying and understanding this boundless, universal act. This has often led to the oversimplification of sexual acts to those of measurable ends like erectile dysfunction in men and vaginal lubrication in women.

In order to simplify this seemingly indescribable task, several authors have conceptualized sexual problems arising from illness as primary, secondary or tertiary

[1–3]. Primary refers to dysfunction that is organic in origin related directly to specific illness effects [2]. All individuals with each particular condition present with similar primary symptoms. Secondary sexual dysfunction relates to the physical changes that cause indirect impairment such as fatigue, weakness and bowel/bladder incontinence [2]. Finally, tertiary sexual dysfunction suggests the psychological stress of illness such as low self-esteem due to changed body image, depression from loss of previous function, and anger or fear of rejection from one's partner or society [2]. Diagnosing primary, secondary or tertiary dysfunction or the combination thereof is complicated but must be attempted as it profoundly affects treatment.

Neurological Disorders

For many, loss of sexual function is the most devastating aspect of neurologic illness. All phases of the sexual response cycle can be affected, from the inability to process sexual stimuli to arousal dysfunction and anorgasmia [3]. Specific to neurologic illness is also heightened sexual function such as spontaneous orgasm in epilepsy or hyperarousal in traumatic brain injury. Hypersexuality is not an increase in sexual needs but characterized more as a general disinhibition [2]. Although neurologic illness extends from the brain to the peripheral nerves, only a select few topics of traumatic brain injury, multiple sclerosis and spinal cord injury will be discussed here. Diabetic neuropathy will be considered later in the endocrine section.

Traumatic Brain Injury

Studies on brain trauma are limited by their subjects' ability to participate related to the biological effects of neuronal trauma and by comorbid mood and pain issues [3]. Many survivors are in the midst of adolescence, just becoming aware of themselves as sensual beings and have yet to have any sexual encounters [2].

Sexual outcomes can be determined globally by the total amount of brain tissue destroyed versus focal deficits associated with the specific area of the brain affected [2, 3]. Globally, arousal may be influenced by verbal and nonverbal communication problems as well as increased impulsivity and altered concentration [2]. Locally, injury to the prefrontal cortex generates apathy with hyposexuality, or less commonly, disinhibition with hypersexuality [2]. Lobar injuries most often produce hyposexuality with the exception of bilateral necrosis of the temporal lobes (Klüver-Bucy syndrome), which causes hypersexuality and hyperorality [2, 3].

Hypothalamic and pituitary damage may be missed at the initial event as basal fractures that injure the pituitary stalk have low detection rates on MRI and CT [3]. Complaints of decreased libido, impotence, and dysmenorrhea may be the first signs of decreased hormone levels [2]. If these endocrine alterations occur early, they may trigger puberty leading to body image struggles and social withdrawal [2]. Although panhypopituitarism is rare in head injury survivors, isolated pituitary deficits, specifically low gonadotropin and low growth hormone, are frequent sequelae [3]. Resulting low testosterone levels hinder sexual well being in both genders as do low growth hormone titers which result in a loss of vitality [3].

Multiple Sclerosis

The etiology of sexual impairment in multiple sclerosis involves both spinal cord lesions and psychologic factors [1, 4]. Primary sexual dysfunction includes altered genital sensation, decreased lubrication, difficulties keeping and maintaining an erection and decreased ability to achieve orgasm [1, 4]. Muscle weakness, spasticity, tremor and sphincter dysfunction comprise the secondary dysfunction [1]. These symptoms may lead to tertiary dysfunction with psychological dissatisfaction and depression. Sexual dysfunction increases with age and disease duration and is associated with anxiety and lower levels of education [1]. Overall, sexual dysfunction contributes to decreased quality of life scores in those living with multiple sclerosis [4].

Spinal Cord Injury

Level and completeness of spinal cord damage determines sexual capacity [3]. Psychogenic erections are lost with high lesions but reflex erections remain intact [3]. For women, those younger at age of trauma were more likely to have sexual encounters after injury [5]. Women's preferred intimate activities after injury included kissing, hugging and touching [5]. Women with complete lower motor neuron dysfunction cannot achieve orgasm with clitoral stimulation, but those with lesions at any level may be able to climax with cervical vibrostimulation [3]. Similar to other neurologic disorders, spasticity, motor restrictions and catheter limitations interfere with sexual activity [5].

Treatment

Because most neurologic illnesses are incurable, sexual dysfunction may be lifelong. Thus, the first step in treatment is for practitioners to be aware of changes in emotional, cognitive, behavioral and functional status after initial diagnosis. Then, frequent assessment of sexual health should occur along with review of other systems. Addressing patients' concerns early on could facilitate discussions with sexual partners that might otherwise be difficult, and thus prevent future problems [2].

Those patients with traumatic brain injury should routinely have hormone levels checked including testosterone and growth hormone as both of these can affect libido, performance and endurance [3]. Supplementation when deficiencies are identified may improve outcomes. Lubricants may also provide some benefit.

An intense research area is the treatment of male erectile dysfunction in spinal cord injury. The mainstay is vacuum tumescence devices which prove satisfactory with few risks [6]. For decades intracavernous penile injections of vasoactive substances including papaverine, phentolamine and prostaglandin have provided excellent erection response rates [6]. Sildenafil is equivalent to intracavernous injections in both efficacy and degree of side effects, but is less successful in men with lower motor neuron injuries [6]. Despite good efficacy, penile implants have decreased in popularity secondary to a consistent 10% complication rate which includes damage to penile tissues rendering them unresponsive to other treatments [3, 6]. Topical and intraurethral agents are only effective a quarter of the time and therefore are not widely used in this population [6].

Endocrine Disorders

Endocrine diseases often diminish sexual function, and sexual disorders may signal endocrine ailments. Most often, these symptoms are treatable once the underlying endocrinopathy is discovered, but too often sexual dysfunction in the endocrine patient is given little attention in clinical practice.

Diabetes

Similar to other disorders, sexual dysfunction in diabetes is multifactorial. Sexual interaction is influenced by decreased energy from suboptimal glycemic control, altered self-image from the obesity related to insulin resistance and the interpersonal difficulties arising from the partner who polices dietary control and glucose monitoring [7]. End-organ damage to neurological and vascular systems contributes to sexual dysfunction, particularly erectile dysfunction, which increases with age and severity of disease and affects up to 75% of men with diabetes [7]. Also associated are poor metabolic control, untreated hypertension and end-organ damage such as nephropathy and retinopathy [7]. Peyronie's disease and ejaculatory problems, including retrograde ejaculation and ejaculatory incompetence secondary to neuropathy, are also more common in this population. Endothelial and smooth muscle dysfunction result from reduced nitric oxide synthase leading to the accumulation of toxic oxygen free radicals which then depletes nitric oxide and damages potassium channels [7]. Pelvic autonomic neuropathy results from similar oxidative stress and nerve hypoxia [7].

Diabetic women's sexual dysfunction is inadequately studied and measurable genital vasocongestion correlates poorly with the subjective sense of arousal [7]. A higher portion of women report loss of orgasmic function and impaired clitoral sexual sensation [7]. Diabetes is a known risk factor for infections, and dyspareunia in diabetic women may be due to chronic vulvar candidiasis [7].

Treatment
Regular screening for sexual problems in patients with diabetes is essential, in part because erectile dysfunction may herald serious cardiac disease. Physical examination and measurement of prolactin and testosterone are indicated if low desire or ejaculation delay is present [7]. The cornerstones of therapy are tight glycemic control and exercise. Phosphodiesterase inhibitors (PD5 inhibitors) are first-line treatment, but should be used with caution as diabetes is a risk factor for heart disease and may mean the patient is taking incompatible cardiac medications. If this class of medication is contraindicated, then transurethral or intracavernosal injections of prostaglandin E1 may be administered [7].

Fewer treatment options currently exist for women. Candidal infections should be adequately treated and vibrostimulation may help in anorgasmia associated with loss of genital sensation [7]. Individual women may respond to phosphodiesterase inhibitors, although in clinical trials PD5 inhibitors failed to separate from placebo.

Androgen Deficiency

Although testosterone is known to influence sexual desire, the mechanism of this affect is largely unknown. Male serum testosterone levels decrease by 1–2% per year, ultimately resulting in testosterone levels in older men that do not differ significantly from the levels of young, healthy males. However, no exact correlation can be made between testosterone levels and depression, erectile dysfunction, symptoms of aging or prostate volume [7]. Interestingly, androgen-deficient males are able to achieve erection from erotic visual stimuli even though spontaneous erection, as in nocturnal penile tumescence, may still be impaired [7].

The diagnosis of androgen insufficiency should be based on 2 separate morning serum testosterone concentrations that are below the level of normal in a young healthy male [7]. Low levels can be caused by primary testicular failure as in uncorrected cryptorchidism, HIV, trauma and radiation therapy [7]. Secondary causes include deficiencies in LH, FSH and GnRH resulting from pituitary tumors, excessive exercise or abuse of opioids, cocaine, alcohol and marijuana [7].

Androgen insufficiency and its subsequent replacement are much more controversial in women as testosterone levels and its effects are even more difficult to measure. Testosterone peaks in the 20s and mean levels fall progressively until the mid 40s when they plateau [8]. Female androgen deficiency syndrome is described in estrogen-replete, testosterone-deficient women as a diminished sense of well-being or dysphoric mood, persistent unexplained fatigue and sexual function changes including decreased libido, diminished sexual receptivity, or reduced pleasure [7–9].

While the definition of female androgen deficiency syndrome appears vague, difficulty still exists in meeting syndromal criteria. Testosterone levels in women vary greatly across the menstrual cycle and with pulsatile diurnal and circannual rhythms [7–9]. Also commercial assays cannot reliably measure the low circulating concentrations seen in women [7–9]. Thus DHEA, a preandrogen released from the ovaries and converted to potent testosterone and dihydroxytestosterone in the peripheral tissues, is often measured concurrently [8, 9]. Low testosterone levels in women are associated with bilateral oopherectomy, panhypopituitarism, oral contraceptive use and COPD [7].

Treatment

Testosterone replacement comes in many forms from tablets and injections to gels and pellets implanted subcutaneously [7]. Androgen replacement is not recommended for men with breast or prostate cancer, elevated prostate-specific antigen levels greater than 3×10^{-12} g/l, hyperviscosity syndrome or uncontrolled heart failure [7]. In men, hematocrit to monitor for erythrocytosis, and prostate-specific antigen levels to screen for prostate cancer should be measured at 3, 6 and 12 months after initiation of androgen therapy. Symptomatic improvements to expect are improved libido but not erectile function or quality of life [7].

Therapeutic androgen use in women is considered off label use as no testosterone products are FDA approved for women. Testosterone administration in premenopausal women is extremely controversial. Transdermal applications and implants are the preferred routes, and free testosterone concentrations should be maintained in the mid- to high-normal range [8, 9]. Reported benefits include improvement in libido, chronic fatigue and sense of well-being [8, 9]. The most commonly reported side effect is hirsuitism, but potential adverse effects include cardiovascular disease, breast cancer, lowered HDL levels and endometrial hyperplasia [8].

Turner's Syndrome

Turner 's syndrome is the partial or total absence of one of the X chromosomes in some or all cells. Women with Turner's syndrome have primary gonadal agenesis resulting in a lack of sex hormones leading to sexual infantilism and impaired fertility. Most girls require estrogen replacement to induce puberty and subsequent lifelong estrogen and progesterone to prevent osteoporosis and cardiac disease [10]. Turner's syndrome patients report a delay in reaching social and sexual milestones, including later sexual debut, fewer partners and less stable intimate relationships [10]. They report less sexual drive, decreased vaginal lubrication and less sexual motivation, often secondary to fear of being reminded of their infertility [10]. However, those in stable relationships report contentment with their sexual life due to a satisfied need for intimacy.

Hyperprolactinemia and Thyroid Disorders

Decreased desire and erectile dysfunction are the most common presenting symptoms in men with hyperprolactinemia [7]. Although amenorrhea and galactorrhea are more bothersome for women, they often complain of decreased libido, diminished lubrication and reduced satisfaction [7]. Prolactin lowers free testosterone levels through inhibitory effects on GnRH secretion with subsequent decreased LH and FSH levels.

Often comorbid with hyperprolactinemia is profound hypothyroidism, which independently causes hypoactive sexual desire, erectile dysfunction and abnormal ejaculation [7]. Men with hypothyroidism have low free testosterone levels as well as decreased sex hormone-binding globulin.

Patients with hyperthyroidism have similar symptoms of decreased libido, premature or delayed ejaculation and erectile dysfunction [9]. However, men have elevated total testosterone concentrations, but low free testosterone levels. Raised sex hormone-binding globulin, and converted testosterone to estrogen can cause gynecomastia [2].

Treatment

Sexual dysfunction in hyperprolactinemia has been treated with moderate success using dopamine agonists such as ropinirole [7]. Surgical removal of the prolactinoma may be necessary. Sexual dysfunction in those with thyroid disease is usually successfully treated by returning patients to a euthyroid state.

Cardiovascular Illness

Heart disease, by virtue of its name seems isolated to one central organ. However, the effects of hypertension and atherosclerosis are systemic, and may cause disease from a bleed in the head to an ulcer on the toe. Sexual dysfunction in patients with atherosclerotic vascular disease may precede quantifiable cardiovascular disease by years. An 11%, 5-year risk of a cardiovascular event in men with erectile dysfunction is comparable to diabetes in terms of cardiovascular risk factors [11]. Unfortunately, treatment of coronary artery disease (CAD) and hypertension can cause even greater sexual impairment resulting in an increased level of medical noncompliance than expected based on other adverse events.

Hypertension

Arterial hypertension is a systemic disorder characterized by altered vascular resistance and cardiac index resulting in high blood pressure. Hypertension may cause endothelial dysfunction by shear stress within the vessel wall leading to reduced vasodilation and subsequent problems with erection and vulvar/vaginal congestion [11]. Although most studies involve men, hypertensive women also have difficulties achieving adequate lubrication and sexual satisfaction [12].

Every patient with erectile dysfunction should have a cardiovascular exam to include palpation of peripheral pulses, observation for signs of peripheral ischemia and measurement of a lipid profile, fasting blood glucose and body mass index.

Treatment

The close association between hypertension and sexual dysfunction may lead one to conclude that adequate blood pressure control could favorably influence the risk and progression of erectile dysfunction or even result in the reversal of symptoms. To the contrary, many anti-hypertensive medications further worsen sexual impairment via specific drug side effects as well as from reduction in pressure in the narrowed pelvic arteries that have adapted to operating in a high pressure system [11, 12]. Beta-blocking agents and thiazide diuretics are notorious for causing erectile dysfunction by increasing the latency to initial erection, reducing the number of erectile reflexes and possibly reducing testosterone levels [13]. Selective beta-1 blockade causes less sexual impairment than the nonselective beta-1 and -2 blocking agents. In contrast, angiotensin receptor blockers seem to improve sexual function with effective blood pressure control by influencing cavernous smooth muscle tone through an effect on the balance between angiotensin II and nitric oxide [11, 13]. Methyldopa, one of the few anti-hypertensives safe in pregnancy, is now prescribed to female hypertensives at all ages and stages of reproductive life [13]. Unfortunately, methyldopa has gained a widespread reputation for disrupting sexual function due to its central adrenergic inhibition [13].

If sexual impairment is forcing the patient to choose between sexual quality of life and long-term cardiovascular health, then perhaps loop diuretics can be substituted for thiazides and angiotensin receptor blockers for angiotensin-converting enzyme inhibitors. Health care providers should end the indiscriminate use of beta-blockers especially in younger hypertensive males. However, if necessary, beta-1 selective blockade should be administered at the lowest effective dose. Phosphodiesterase-5 (PDE-5) inhibitors, now often first-line in treating ED, may reduce systolic and diastolic blood pressure by 7–10 mm Hg in a nondose-dependent manner without any evidence of significant reflex tachycardia [11]. Thus, medications such as sildenafil are considered relatively safe in the hypertensive patient with a baseline blood pressure of more than 90/60 mm Hg [11].

Vascular Disease

Erectile dysfunction is found in 39% of men with CAD and 56% of smoking cardiac patients [14]. Women with diagnosed CAD have statistically significant decreases in

Female Sexual Function Index scores for desire, orgasm, arousal and number of intercourse episodes [15]. While revascularization of the pelvic and lower extremity vessels may improve erectile function, aortoiliac and femoral bypass may injure the hypogastric nerve and artery thereby worsening erectile dysfunction [13].

While exercise is encouraged in these patients, misconceptions remain as to the risk of triggering a cardiovascular event by sexual activity [16]. The workload during coitus and orgasm is modest; metabolic cost is 2.5–3.5 metabolic equivalents of task (equivalent to walking briskly up two flights of stairs) with a mean blood pressure of 162/89 [15]. Less than 1% of myocardial infarctions and 0.6% of sudden cardiac deaths appear related to sexual activity [11, 15]. Caution regarding sexual activity should be reserved for those who have a severely diminished exercise capacity secondary to chest pain and/ or dyspnea.

Treatment

Healthcare providers should be aware of the strong bidirectional association between erectile dysfunction and cardiovascular illness. While taking a medical history, sexual dysfunction should be elicited along with other vascular risk factors. Risk of erectile dysfunction should be disclosed as a potential complication before any vascular surgery involving the aortic, iliac or femoral arteries [14].

Although no treatment substitutes for regular exercise, a low-fat diet and smoking cessation, several medications have been shown to be safe in this population. PDE-5 inhibitors cause no increase in rates of myocardial infarction or death, and may actually improve exercise time in heart failure patients, and positively effect regression of right ventricular hypertrophy [15]. However, they are absolutely contraindicated in the many cardiovascular patients taking nitrates (e.g. nitroglycerin) and used with caution with coadministration of alpha-adrenoreceptor blockers (e.g. doxazosin) [11, 15]. Organic nitrates increase the production of cyclic GMP while PDE-5 inhibitors prevent its breakdown, which while improving initiation and maintenance of penile erection, can lead to vasodilation and profound hypotension [15]. Hypotension in those on alpha-adrenoreceptor blockers for prostatic hyperplasia is less significant than initially assumed but coadministration with PDE-5 inhibitors should be reserved for those under close medical monitoring with no other available alternatives [11].

Stroke

Sexual dysfunction in stroke patients represents a complex interplay of organic and psychological factors. The mean decline of sexual performance after stroke is 83% [17]. However, sexual problems are common in patients with comorbid prestroke vascular disorders including diabetes, hypertension and cardiac disease. Stroke survivors are often administered cardiovascular medications (such as beta-blockers) further worsening sexual dysfunction [18, 19]. Decreased libido and satisfaction correlate with the existence and severity of depression [17]. Similar to other neurologic illnesses, sexual function in stroke patients is also affected by difficulties with self-care and potentially unattractive behaviors such as drooling and incontinence [17, 18]. Fear of relapse experienced by both patient and partner leads to decreased sexual activity [16]. But more importantly, partners often discourage sex due to the belief that a sexual life only belongs to healthy people and harbor lack of excitation or even disgust at the notion of having sexual intercourse with the disabled patient [16].

Although no consensus exists, poststroke sexual dysfunction is believed to be dependent on specific injured brain regions that control libido and sexual behavior [18]. Hypersexuality can manifest in patients with lacunar infarcts in the thalamus and frontolimbic regions [3]. Sexual impairment from left hemisphere lesions may be explained by reduced ability to communicate intimately with the partner or to initiate and maintain sexual interest and arousal mediated through the left frontal lobe [17]. Temporal lobe injury leading to poststroke emotional incontinence may result in decreased sexual activity [18]. Libido and erection may require activation within the cortical and limbic structures which are regulated by the right hemisphere's ability to recognize emotional stimuli [18]. Patients with right temporal lobe dysfunction have increased serum prolactin, LH and FSH levels leading to decreased libido and impotence [17]. Finally the autonomic disarray commonly observed in right hemispheric stroke patients may play a role in erectile dysfunction and problems with ejaculation through the complex sympathetic and parasympathetic interplay of smooth and skeletal fibers, and glandular and endothelial cells [18].

Treatment
A large percentage of patients who attend rehabilitation programs can spontaneously regain erectile function within months of injury [3]. Early attention to nutrition, including tube feeding, is essential in preventing reduction of adipocyte-secreted leptin, which helps regulate gonadotropin secretion [3].

Pelvic Disease

The pelvis is a funnel-shaped compartment housing the genitourinary organs supported in an interconnected neuromuscular web. Because of this organization of interrelated muscle, and sympathetic and parasympathetic fibers, dysfunction in one compartment of the pelvis can disrupt performance in another area. Sexual health can be influenced by diseased sexual organs, incontinence or surgery anywhere in the pelvic region. Although a natural condition in most women's lives, pregnancy may also cause bowel, bladder and sexual dysfunction.

Proctectomy

Proctectomy is most often performed to treat rectal cancer in older patients but has been used in younger people with inflammatory bowel disease and familial adenomatous polyposis [20]. Most women however are in midlife and already experiencing preoperative female sexual dysfunction secondary to physiologic and hormonal changes associated with reduced estrogen. Deep pelvic dissection may injure sympathetic nerves resulting in reduced vaginal lubrication [20].

Although both men and women experience sexual limitations, males report more distress even a year after surgery [21]. Impotence is related to transection of the inferior hypogastric plexus, whereas ejaculatory dysfunction results from disruption of the superior hypogastric plexus [20]. Sexual dysfunction is increased in both genders when surgery is combined with radiotherapy in advanced tumors. Rectal sphincter-sparing surgery causes the least sexual dysfunction compared to laparoscopic-assisted surgery or the anterior/abdominoperineal approach [20, 21].

Treatment

Since less than 9% of patients postoperatively recall discussing potential sexual outcomes preoperatively, clinicians must make extra efforts to explain the myriad of difficulties that can occur so that patients can make the most informed decisions about their care [19]. Topical agents are available for decreased vaginal lubrication and both penile and clitoral tumescence devices exist to aid genital congestion [20].

Urinary Incontinence and Overactive Bladder Syndrome

Urinary incontinence can deter women from sexual fulfillment from fear of urine leakage during the sexual act and embarrassment from odor and dampness. They report worse body image, more medical conditions and worse mental health. Female Sexual Function Index scores in premenopausal women are inversely related to the number of incontinence pads used [22]. Interestingly, many older women remain sexually active regardless of their continence status [23]. This may be due to better body image in women over the age of 50. However, even in this subset, older women report less sexual activity if they have nocturnal incontinence or experience large amounts of urine loss [22].

Women with overactive bladders may have urinary incontinence but the syndrome is defined by urgency, frequency and nocturia [24]. Due to their voiding symptoms, these patients become house-bound, drink less fluid and avoid visiting places without a bathroom [23]. They report increased sexual problems with age and associated with a history of urinary tract infections. Women with overactive bladder symptoms avoid sexual encounters due to urgency to void during intercourse, suprapubic pain and vulvodynia [23]. As with urinary incontinence, younger women think of themselves as less sexually attractive secondary to the need to wear pads to bed.

Hysterectomy

Although hysterectomy is the most frequently performed nonobstetric surgical procedure in the US, only recently have effects on sexual function been studied [25]. Women tend to undergo hysterectomy with salping-oopherectomy for excessive vaginal bleeding and find an improvement in a variety of symptoms including pelvic pain, dyspareunia, fatigue and premenstrual mood symptoms [25]. While most women can expect unchanged or improved sexual function, some report increased vaginal dryness or decreased sexual desire with bilateral oopherectomy [26]. However, due to the fact that women describe unchanged, worsened and improved sexual function with ovary-sparing hysterectomy, difficulty exists in predicting a specific outcome for an individual patient. The cervix may play a significant role in sexual satisfaction, and women report a decrease in orgasmic ability after undergoing abdominal hysterectomy versus those who had a supracervical hysterectomy [25]. Most women seem to recover from sexual dysfunction 2 years after surgery independent of the procedure performed [25].

Treatment of Pelvic Disease

Patient education prior to any pelvic surgery regarding possible sexual outcomes helps to mitigate the negative side effects of these procedures [25]. Many women after having a gynecologic cancer experience their bodies as having failed them and become distracted by a scar or mourn the loss of genital arousal. Some patients have found mindfulness therapy of 'staying in the moment' and avoiding negative distractions helps to focus them on the actual sexual encounter instead of unpleasant thoughts [27]. Pelvic floor strengthening exercises may improve continence and sexual function, but more invasive procedures such as abdominal uterine suspension may be necessary.

Pregnancy

Beliefs about sexuality as well as physical and emotional changes come into play during pregnancy. Coitus duration decreases over the length of pregnancy likely due to the unfounded fear that intercourse may hurt the mother or baby and/or cause premature labor [28]. Women also report deterioration in body image as they gain weight. Although vaginal dryness improves, especially in the last trimester, patients frequently report dyspareunia and decline in orgasm incidence as pregnancy progresses [25]. Also, anatomical changes compel couples to attempt sexual positions with which they may not be as comfortable.

Not only pregnancy, but mode of delivery may have lasting effects on sexual function. Even 6 months after delivery, primiparous women who delivered vaginally by mediolateral episiotomy report decreased levels of desire, arousal, lubrication, orgasm, and satisfaction, as well as increased dyspareunia compared to women who deliver by cesarean section [29]. Low desire may be due to the new mothers' association of pain upon penetration. Women who deliver vaginally have weakened pelvic floors and may also have discomfort secondary to cystoceles and rectoceles. While vaginal delivery is preferred over cesarean section for the health of mother and child, women who deliver vaginally should be warned of possible sexual side effects and instructed in Kegel exercises for pelvic floor strengthening early in the postpartum period.

Prostate Illness

Benign Prostatic Hypertrophy

Benign prostatic hypertrophy is the most common cause of lower urinary tract symptoms (LUTS) such as nocturia, frequency, urgency, dysuria, hesitancy and overflow incontinence. LUTS is strongly associated with erectile and ejaculatory dysfunction independent of age, medical comorbidities and lifestyle factors [30]. The exact pathophysiological mechanism is unknown, but the common pathway seems to be smooth muscle myopathy due to loss of smooth muscle cells and subsequent collagen deposition [30].

Treatment

Unfortunately, the treatment for LUTS/benign prostatic hypertrophy may accentuate sexual dysfunction. The alpha-1 blocker tamsulosin causes decreased ejaculatory volume and the 5-reductase inhibitor finasteride worsens erectile and ejaculatory dysfunction. Although surgical intervention such as transurethral resection of the prostate may improve certain aspects of sexual function including erectile function and painful ejaculation, it may still cause erectile and ejaculatory problems. The combination of a PDE-5 inhibitor and an alpha-1 blocker (such as doxasozin) has been shown to improve sexual performance.

Radical Prostatectomy

Radical prostatectomy remains the most common treatment of clinically localized prostate cancer in men with at least a 10-year life expectancy. Careful patient selection and bilateral nerve sparing, or preservation of the neurovascular bundles, are the major determinants of postoperative erectile function [31]. Unfortunately, permanent impotency is the reality for most patients secondary to tissue damage induced by poor corporeal oxygenation leading to penile fibrosis [31].

Treatment
Treatment focuses on prophylaxis aimed at improving early postoperative corporeal filling. Administration of a PDE-5 inhibitor facilitates the occurrence of nocturnal erections which are believed to have a natural protective role on the baseline function of the corpus cavernosa. Patients either not responding to or who cannot use oral PDE-5 inhibitors may be candidates for intraurethral or intracorporeal administration of alprostadil [31].

Other Illnesses

Breast Cancer

Although breast cancer itself is not associated with sexual dysfunction, the surgical, radiological and hormonal treatment for breast neoplasm is. Women undergoing radical mastectomy experience greater sexual dysfunction than those receiving breast-conserving therapy [32]. This is due in part to the tertiary or psychological sexual dysfunction where partners of lumpectomy patients initiate sexual activity more frequently than partners of mastectomy patients [33]. The less women perceive their partner to be bothered by the scar, the higher they rate their first postsurgical experience [30].

The secondary sexual dysfunction of fatigue, weight loss, alopecia and nausea associated with chemotherapy often affects a woman's sense of femininity and sexuality. Women undergoing chemotherapy report a decrease in sexual interest and activity as well as dyspareunia [30]. Due to immunosuppression, many patients complain of opportunistic infections of yeast, genital herpes and vaginal warts [34]. These sexually transmitted diseases, as well as the cytotoxic waste excreted in bodily fluids further complicate interpersonal relationships by making the sex a risky undertaking for the partner involved [31].

Postmenopausal women report less vaginal dryness, decreased libido and reduced breast sensitivity with the endocrine therapies which can induce abrupt ovarian failure than women of reproductive age [30]. As survival rates in breast cancer increase, more women are maintained on systemic adjuvant therapy for 5–10 years following diagnosis [29, 31]. This means that initially tolerable sexual difficulties in the face of fighting the disease may become unbearable as women try to resume their previous lifestyles.

Treatment
As often happens with malignancy, issues of survival overshadow concerns with quality of life. However, expressions of sexuality can remain an intimate form of

communication that relieves suffering throughout the cancer process [31]. Vaginal lubricants and estrogen creams help reduce vaginal dryness [30]. Most oncologists debate the safety of estrogen and testosterone replacement therapy due to their possible systemic effects in hormone receptor-positive neoplasms. Transvaginal estrogens, such as Estring, have limited systemic absorption because they bypass first pass metabolism, and they also have a low incidence of deep venous thrombosis. Alternative treatments for vasomotor symptoms include vitamin E and venlafaxine, although serotonin and norepinephrine reuptake inhibitors may cause more sexual dysfunction [30].

Rheumatoid Arthritis

Rheumatoid arthritis is a chronic autoimmune inflammatory disease that affects all joints leading to various degrees of disability. Patients complain of difficulty performing sexual acts secondary to hip and knee immobility [35]. Sexual desire is dampened by pain, negative body image, fatigue, morning stiffness and dyspareunia due to vaginal dryness associated with Sjögren's disease [33]. Because of joint immobility, women are not regularly screened for genital tract abnormalities such as infection, uterine prolapse and Bartholin's cysts, which may further reduce sexual satisfaction.

Psoriasis

Psoriasis is a chronic inflammatory skin disease that may also affect the joints, but patient's sexual dysfunction appears to stem more from physical disfigurement [36]. Those patients who saw themselves as sexually undesirable tended to be older with higher levels of plaque desquamation [34]. Reduction in clinical severity by intense treatment for psoriasis leads to improved sexual functioning.

End-Stage Renal Disease

Although dialysis improves many symptoms of end-stage renal disease including pruritis from uremia, dyspnea from fluid overload and altered mentation from electrolyte disarray, many patients continue to experience sexual dysfunction. Fatigue from anemia of chronic disease, hyperprolactinemia, hyperparathyroidism and zinc deficiency lead to reduced libido, impotence and decreased frequency of sexual relations [37]. Since most renal failure in the US is caused by diabetes, hypertension and atherosclerosis, patients must not only suffer with these comorbid illnesses, but also with the sexually impairing medications used to treat them.

Table 1. Medication effects on sexual function [40]

Drug class	Phase of sexual cycle			Other
	desire	arousal	orgasm	
Chemotherapeutic agents	×	×		
Triglyceride-lowering agents		×		
Antifungals	×	×		
Histamine receptor (H2) blockers		×		
Proton pump inhibitors				painful nocturnal erections
Nonsteroidal anti-inflammatory agents	×	×		
Narcotics	×	×	×	
Opioid antagonists			×	
Weight loss agents		×	×	
Nonselective beta-antagonists		×		
Central alpha-adrenergic agonists			×	
Thiazide diuretics		×		
Oral contraceptives	×	×		
Immunosuppressants	×			
Antiepileptics			×	

Of note, almost any illness may affect sexual function through primary organic symptoms, secondary symptoms such as effects on energy level, or tertiary psychological sequelae.

Medication-Induced Dysfunction

Oral Contraceptives

Eighty percent of women born since 1945 have used oral contraception as their means of birth control and over the decades some have reported diminished sexual interest, arousal, suppression of female-initiated sexual activity and decreased frequency of sexual intercourse (table 1) [38]. Exogenous estrogen and progesterone are known to decrease circulating levels of androgens by direct inhibition of androgen production in the ovaries and by marked increase in the hepatic synthesis of sex hormone-binding globulin [36]. This in turn leads to low circulating levels of bioavailable testosterone, which many believe is involved in sexual dysfunction. Long-term, even permanent, effects on sexual health may occur as sex hormone-binding globulin levels remain elevated over baseline even 6 months after discontinuing oral contraceptives [36].

Immunosuppressants

Although significant improvements in health may be expected with organ transplantation, lifelong treatment with immunosuppressants may pose quality of life challenges. Many complain of feeling physically unattractive due to obesity, fluid retention, and hirsuitism [39]. Often, the key immunosuppressant administered is a systemic corticosteroid which may cause the problems mentioned above plus the classic buffalo hump, cushionoid facies and depression. This all leads to low sexual self-esteem, making patients uncomfortable seeking sexual pleasure and asking another to help satisfy sexual needs [37]. In addition, many transplant recipients have experienced diabetes, renal failure and/or hypertension, which may cause significant sexual dysfunction or occur with treatments for these disorders.

Antiepileptics

Sexual dysfunction has been linked to anticonvulsants that induce the hepatic p450 system such as phenytoin, carbamazepine, phenobarbital and primidone [3]. These antiepileptics progressively increase sex hormone-binding globulin, and thus decrease free testosterone. Valproic acid increases estradiol levels in both genders as well as causes weight gain and possible mood disturbance [3]. Male epileptic patients treated with these medications complain of erectile and ejaculatory dysfunction while their female counterparts report delayed orgasm [2]. Sexual effects may be avoided by using enzyme- neutral medications such as gabapentin, lamotrigine, levitiracetam and pregabalin [3]. Men may benefit from treatment with testosterone together with an aromatase inhibitor which will reduce conversion of androgen to estrogen [3].

Conclusions

As the population ages, patients may live with their chronic illnesses for years. Thus quality of life becomes ever more important and one of its best measures is sexual health. The media and our youth-obsessed society might confine sexuality to the young and healthy, but patients of all ages and abilities still engage in sexual intimacy as a means to connect with their partners as well as to enhance their sense of well-being. While life-threatening illness often precludes the discussion of sexual health, practitioners still consistently fall short with regard to inquiring about patients' sexual difficulties once their patients have stabilized. This is in part due to the health care team's lack of knowledge about sexual dysfunction and treatment, and the discomfort with discussing a sensitive topic. Also, in the world of 15-min office visits, physicians tend to define patients by their disease entity and not as a multi-faceted sexual being. Thus, the first step in treating sexual dysfunction is becoming aware of its association with almost every diseased organ system. Patients repeatedly report their relief and willingness to discuss sexual problems when the topic is broached by the health care provider. By diagnosing and treating sexual dysfunction, practitioners will not only help to enhance patients' quality of life but also make their complicated, and often painful, treatment regimens more bearable.

References

1 Demirkiran M, Sarica Y, Uguz S, Yerdelen D, Aslan K: Multiple sclerosis patients with and without sexual dysfunction: are there any differences. Mult Scler 2006;12:209–214.

2 Aloni R, Katz S: A review on the effect of traumatic brain injury on the human sexual response. Brain Inj 2007;13:269–280.

3 Rees PM, Fowler CJ, Maas CP: Sexual dysfunction in men and women with neurological disorders. Lancet 2007;369:512–525.

4 Nortvedt M, Riise T, Frugård J, Mohn J, Bakke A, Skår A, Nyland H, Glad S, Myhr K: Prevalence of bladder, bowel and sexual problems among multiple sclerosis patients two to five years after diagnosis. Mult Scler 2007;13:106–112.

5 Black K, Sipski M, Strauss S: Sexual satisfaction and sexual drive in spinal cord injured women. J Spinal Cord Med 1998;21:240–244.

6 DeForge D, Blackmer J, Garrity C, Yazdi F, Cronin V, Barrowman N, Fang M, Mamaladze V, Zhang L, Sampson M, Moher D: Male erectile dysfunction following spinal cord injury: a systematic review. Spinal Cord 2006;44:465–473.

7 Bhasin S, Enzlin P, Coviello A, Basson R: Sexual dysfunction in men and women with endocrine disorders. Lancet 2007;369:597–611.

8 Burger H, Papalia M: A clinical update on female androgen insufficiency-testosterone testing and treatment in women presenting with low sexual desire. Sex Health 2006;3:73–78.

9 Traish A, Guay A, Spark R: Are the endocrine society's clinical practice guidelines on androgen therapy in women misguided? A commentary. J Sex Med 2007;4:1223–1235.

10 Rolstad S, Möller A, Bryman I, Boman U: Sexual functioning and partner relationships in women with Turner syndrome: some empirical data and theoretical considerations regarding sexual desire. J Sex Marital Ther 2007;33:231–247.

11 Refflemann T, Kloner R: Sexual dysfunction in hypertensive patients receiving treatment. Vasc Health Risk Manage 2006;2:447–455.

12 Okeahialam B, Obeka N: Sexual dysfunction in female hypertensives. J Natl Med Assoc 2006;98: 638–640.

13 Jassim Al Kaja K, Sequeira R, Al Damanhori H, Mathur V: Anti-hypertensive drug-associated sexual dysfunction: a prescription analysis-based study. Pharmacoepidemiol Drug Saf 2003;12:203–212.

14 Falkensammer J, Hakaim A, Falkensammer C, Broderick G, Crook J, Heckman M, Oldenburg A, Hugl B: Prevalence of erectile dysfunction in vascular surgery patients. Vasc Med 2007;12:17–22.

15 Kaya C, Yilmaz G, Nurkalem Z, Ilktac A, Karaman M: Sexual function in women with coronary artery disease: a preliminary study. Int J Impot Res 2007; 19:326–329.

16 Kiowski W, Brunner H, Schalcher C: Sex, the heart, and heart failure. Semin Cardiovasc Vasc Anesth 2006;109:256–258.

17 Giaquinto S, Buzzelli S, Fancesco L, Nolfe G: Evaluation of sexual changes after stroke. J Clin Psychiatry 2003;64:302–307.

18 Kimura M, Murata Y, Shimoda K, Robinson R: Sexual dysfunction following stroke. Compr Psychiatry 2001;42:217–222.

19 Pistoia F, Govoni S, Boselli C: Sex after stroke: A CNS only dysfunction? Pharmacol Res 2006;54:11–18.

20 Izanec J, Nagle D: Impact of proctectomy on continence and sexual function in women. Am J Gastroenterol 2006;101:618–624.

21 Schmidt C, Bestmann B, Küchler T, Kremer B: Factors influencing sexual function in patients with rectal cancer. Int J Impot Res 2005;17:231–238.

22 Aslan G, Köseoğlu H, Sadik Ö, Gimen S, Cihan A, Esen A: Sexual function in women with urinary incontinence. Int J Impot Res 2005;17:248–251.

23 Tannenbaum C, Corcos J, Assalian P: The relationship between sexual activity and urinary incontinence in older women. J Am Geriatr Soc 2006;54:1220–1224.

24 Kim Y, Seo J, Yoon H: The effect of overactive bladder syndrome on the sexual quality of life in Korean young and middle aged women. Int J Impot Res 2005;17:158–163.

25 Carlson K: Outcomes of hysterectomy. Clin Obstet Gynecol 1997;40:939–946.
26 Bradford A, Meston C: Sexual outcomes and satisfaction with hysterectomy: influence of patient education. J Sex Med 2007;4:106–114.
27 Brotto L, Heiman J: Mindfulness in sex therapy: applications for women with sexual difficulties following gynecologic cancer. Sex Relationship Ther 2007;22:5–11.
28 Gökyildiz Ş, Beji N: The effects of pregnancy on sexual life. J Sex Marital Ther 2005;31:201–215.
29 Baksu B, Davas I, Agar E, Akyol A, Varolan A: The effect of mode of delivery on postpartum sexual functioning in primiparous women. Int Urogynecol J 2007;18:401–406.
30 Rosen R: Update on the relationship between sexual dysfunction and lower urinary tract symptoms/benign prostatic hyperplasia. Curr Opin Urol 2006;16:11–19.
31 Briganti A, Salonia A, Gallina A, Chun F, Karakiewicz P, Graefen M, Huland H, Rigatti P, Montorsi F: Management of erectile dysfunction after radical prostatectomy in 2007. World J Urol 2007;25:143–148.
32 Stead M: Sexual dysfunction after treatment for gynaecologic and breast malignancies. Curr Opin Obstet Gynecol 2003;15:57–61.
33 Wimberly S, Carver C, Laurenceau J, Harris S, Antoni M: Perceived partner reactions to diagnosis and treatment of breast cancer: impact on psychosocial and psychosexual adjustment. J Consult Clin Psychol 2005;73:300–311.
34 Hordern A: Intimacy and sexuality for the woman with breast cancer. Cancer Nurs 2000;23:230–236.
35 Abdel-Nasser A, Ali E: Determinants of sexual disability and dissatisfaction in female patients with rheumatoid arthritis. Clin Rheumatol 2006;25:822–830.
36 Sampogna F, Gisondi P, Tabolli S, Abeni D: Impairments of sexual life in patients with psoriasis. Dermatology 2007;214:144–150.
37 Soykan A, Boztas H, Kutlay S, Ince E, Nergizoglu G, Dileköz AY, Berksun O: Do sexual dysfunctions get better during dialysis? Results of a six-month prospective follow-up study from Turkey. Int J Impot Res 2005;17:359–363.
38 Panzer C, Wise S, Fantini G, Kang D, Murarriz R, Guay A, Goldstein I: Impact of oral contraceptives on sex hormone-binding globulin and androgen levels: a retrospective study in women with sexual dysfunction. J Sex Med 2006;3:104–113.
39 Muehrer R, Keller M, Powwattana A, Pornchaikate A: Sexuality among women recipients of a pancreas and kidney transplant. West J Nurs Res 2006;28:137–150.
40 Abramowiez M: Drugs that cause sexual dysfunction: an update. Med Lett 1992;34:73–78.

Anita Clayton, MD
University of Virginia, Department of Psychiatry and Neurobehavioral Sciences
PO Box 800623
Charlottesville, VA 22908 (USA)
Tel. +1 434 924 5408, Fax +1 434 924 5149, E-Mail ahc8v@virginia.edu

Balon R (ed): Sexual Dysfunction. The Brain-Body Connection.
Adv Psychosom Med. Basel, Karger, 2008, vol 29, pp 89–106

The Impact of Mental Illness on Sexual Dysfunction

Zvi Zemishlany · Abraham Weizman

Geha Mental Health Center, Petah-Tikva, and Sackler Faculty of Medicine,
Tel-Aviv University, Tel Aviv, Israel

Abstract

Sexual dysfunction is prevalent among psychiatric patients and may be related to both the psychopathology and the pharmacotherapy. The negative symptoms of schizophrenia limit the capability for interpersonal and sexual relationships. The first-generation antipsychotics cause further deterioration in erectile and orgasmic function. Due to their weak antagonistic activity at D2 receptors, second-generation antipsychotics are associated with fewer sexual side effects, and thus may provide an option for schizophrenia patients with sexual dysfunction. Depression and anxiety are a cause for sexual dysfunction that may be aggravated by antidepressants, especially selective serotonin reuptake inhibitors (SSRIs). SSRI-induced sexual dysfunction may be overcome by lowering doses, switching to an antidepressant with low propensity to cause sexual dysfunction (bupropion, mirtazapine, nefazodone, reboxetine), addition of 5HT2 antagonists (mirtazapine, mianserin) or coadministration of 5-phosphodiesterase inhibitors. Eating disorders and personality disorders, mainly borderline personality disorder, are also associated with sexual dysfunction. Sexual dysfunction in these cases stems from impaired interpersonal relationships and may respond to adequate psychosexual therapy. It is mandatory to identify the specific sexual dysfunction and to treat the patients according to his/her individual psychopathology, current pharmacotherapy and interpersonal relationships.

Proper sexual functioning is one of the most important components of quality of life and of maintaining a satisfying intimate relationship. Sexual dysfunction is a common phenomenon in the general population, affecting an estimated 43% of women and 31% of men in the US [1]. The most common dysfunction amongst women is decrease in sexual desire reported by approximately a third of the women. The most common dysfunctions amongst men are erectile dysfunction (ED; mainly in older age) and premature ejaculation. Despite the importance and high prevalence of sexual dysfunction, most sufferers do not seek help either due to feeling of embarrassment or because they do not view it as a medical problem [1, 2].

Table 1. Assessment of sexual dysfunction

Premorbid sexual function
Primary psychiatric disorder
Comorbid psychiatric disorders
Comorbid physical illnesses
Psychotropic medications
Concomitant medications

The prevalence of sexual dysfunctions is higher in persons with mental disorders, particularly those treated with psychotropic medications. For instance, sexual dysfunction has been reported in as many as 30–60% of patients with schizophrenia treated with antipsychotic medications [2], up to 78% of individuals with depression treated with antidepressants [3–5], and up to 80% in patients suffering from anxiety disorders [6, 7].

An evaluation of a sexual dysfunction in psychiatric patients should take into consideration primary sexual functioning, the psychiatric disorders, physical diseases and the various medications (table 1). Sexual dysfunction may be comorbid with, and often a first sign of many physical illnesses and contributes significantly to reduction in quality of life. Awareness of the prevalence and of the hypothesized mechanisms of sexual dysfunctions in psychiatric patients would improve the attitude of the treating physicians towards sexual difficulties in those patients and result in increased compliance with treatment on the patients' part.

Neurotransmitters and Sexual Functioning

Sexual functioning is mediated and influenced, in a complex manner, by endocrine factors, neurotransmitters and neuropeptides.

The endocrine factors include androgens, estrogens, progesterone, prolactin, oxytocin, cortisol and pheromones. Neurotransmitters that are implicated in sexual functioning, mainly dopamine, serotonin and epinephrine, are also implicated in the pathophysiology of the major psychiatric disorders and in their pharmacological treatment.

Dopamine

Studies in humans and animals have suggested that the central dopaminergic system is involved in all components of male sexual behavior: desire, erection, orgasm and satisfaction [8, 9]. Dopaminergic agonists such as L-dopa, apomorphine, amantadine, bupropion and amphetamines have been reported to arouse sexual behavior while central dopaminergic blockers, like antipsychotics, suppress sexual functioning in both animals and humans.

Serotonin

Findings from animal studies suggest that 5-HT may facilitate, inhibit, or have no effect on sexual behavior, depending on which serotonin receptor subtype is involved. Studies on the effect of antidepressants on human sexual functioning suggest that activation of the 5-HT2 receptor impairs all stages of sexual response in males and females [8, 9]. Paroxetine, an SSRI, has been shown to be also a nitric oxide synthase inhibitor, and may diminish nitric oxide levels and function [10].

Epinephrine

Epinephrine inhibits erectile response in men, while blocking α_1-receptors stimulates erection. By contrast, in women epinephrine facilitates vasocongestion while suppression of adrenergic activity impairs sexual arousal and orgasm [9].

Norepinephrine

Norepinephrine levels increase during sexual arousal in both men and women. The few studies that were done so far on this subject suggest that increasing the level of norepinephrine may facilitate erectile response in men [for review, see 9].

Acetylcholine

Acetylcholine facilitates penile erection via the relaxation of smooth muscles of the corpus cavernosum. The role of acetylcholine in female vasocongestion is unclear [9].

Sexual Dysfunctions in Schizophrenia Patients

Patients suffering from schizophrenia (about 1% of the population) are prone to experience sexual dysfunction as a part of the nature of the disease. The premorbid personality of these patients is often schizoid or schizotypal with few interpersonal relationships and lack of sexual experience. Negative symptoms of the disorder, such as anhedonia, avolition and blunted affect related to hypodopaminergic activity in the frontal cortex, severely harm the ability to enjoy sexual life. In addition, these patients face difficulties in establishing relationships due to recurrent psychotic episodes, obesity and low self esteem. Schizophrenia patients are regularly treated with antipsychotics whose common mechanism (at least for the typical antipsychotics) is blockade of postsynaptic D2 dopaminergic receptors.

Few studies have investigated the prevalence of sexual dysfunction amongst schizophrenia patients. The available data focus mainly on dysfunction in males. In one of the first studies, Kotin et al. [11] have shown that 60% of schizophrenia patients treated with thioridazine exhibit sexual dysfunction (35% ED) compared with 25% of patients treated with other typical antipsychotics. Other studies have also found that the prevalence of sexual dysfunction in schizophrenia patients, maintained on first-generation antipsychotics, is 37–54% [12, 13]. Aizenberg et al. [14] examined two groups of treated and untreated male schizophrenia patients and found that both groups reported high prevalence of sexual dysfunction compared to a healthy control group. Untreated patients reported diminished sexual desire and poor sexual performance. Antipsychotic treatment was associated with further deterioration in erection, orgasm and satisfaction with sexual functioning. The antipsychotic-induced ED interferes with the adherence to the medication regime and results in recurrences of psychotic episodes and rehospitalizations.

A recent study assessed sexual dysfunction in men and women with schizophrenia, using a self-completed, gender-specific questionnaire, and compared the results to the general population [15]. At least one sexual dysfunction was reported by 82% of men and 96% of women with schizophrenia. Male patients reported less desire for sex (52 vs. 12%), ED (52 vs. 9%) and more frequently had no sexual intercourse or masturbation (27 vs. 0%). Female patients reported less enjoyment than the control group (46 vs. 5%). Sexual dysfunction in female patients was associated with negative schizophrenia symptoms and general psychopathology. In both men and women there was no association between sexual dysfunction and type of antipsychotic medication. The results of this study, although interesting, are limited due to a small sample size and usage of a self-reporting questionnaire not previously validated. Moreover, few of the patients but most controls had a partner. It was not possible to separate the effects of the illness from those of the medication on sexual dysfunction.

Attempts to treat sexual dysfunction in patients maintained on typical antipsychotics by coadministration of dopaminergic agonists did not bring about the desirable results. Furthermore, the addition of L-dopa may exacerbate psychotic states in schizophrenia patients [16]. Apomorphine causes severe nausea and has, therefore, minimal utility as a therapeutic agent [17]. Coadministration of 100 mg/day of amantadine, a dopamine reuptake inhibitor, for 6 weeks in an open-label study showed some statistically significant improvement in sexual function scores, but insufficient clinically [18]. However, the degree to which placebo effects contributed to the improved sexual function in this open-label study cannot be disregarded. In a double-blind placebo-controlled crossover preliminary study in 10 antipsychotic-treated male schizophrenia outpatients, selegiline (L-deprenyl) 15 mg/day was coadministered with the regular antipsychotic treatment. Selegiline is a selective monoamine oxidase B inhibitor. In low doses (up to 15 mg/day), it selectively inhibits the oxidation of dopamine and phenylethylamine [19]. Selegiline was not found to be effective in improving any domain of sexual functioning in spite of a significant decrease in prolactin levels [20].

The introduction of the new atypical antipsychotics carried expectations for fewer sexual side effects. Atypical antipsychotics as a group have a number of potential advantages over typical antipsychotics in minimizing sexual dysfunction. They display stronger 5-HT2a receptor affinity, relative to D2 receptor affinity and comprise a lower risk for plasma prolactin elevation as well as for extrapyramidal symptoms, which may interfere with sexual function. Atypical antipsychotics have less effect on peripheral cholinergic and α_1-adrenergic receptors involved in sexual function [21].

Hummer et al. [22] conducted a prospective investigation of 100 schizophrenia patients treated with clozapine and 53 patients treated with haloperidol. They found no statistically significant difference between haloperidol and clozapine with regard to their propensity to induce sexual side effects. However, in a similar comparison in male outpatients with chronic schizophrenia, Aizenberg et al. [23] found that, compared to first-generation antipsychotics, maintenance therapy with clozapine may be associated with a better orgasmic function, enjoyment of sex and sexual satisfaction. It seems that the beneficial properties of clozapine (fewer extrapyramidal symptoms, no prolactin elevation) were offset by its relatively greater antiadrenergic and anticholinergic activity, thereby explaining the absence of significant differences in sexual function as regards desire and erectile function [21].

Among atypical antipsychotics, risperidone has been associated with the most substantial changes in serum prolactin concentration and has been found to produce dose-dependent increases in serum prolactin that are comparable to those produced by first-generation antipsychotics [24]. An international trial showed that 4–8 mg of risperidone resulted in sexual side effects comparable to those of haloperidol [25].

In recent years, there has been cumulative clinical evidence that the atypical antipsychotics olanzapine, quetiapine and ziprasidone, which do not bring about a massive blockade of dopamine transmission, cause less disturbances in sexual functioning and may have an advantage over other antipsychotics.

Bitter et al. [26] examined sexual functioning among schizophrenia patients treated for the first time. Five hundred and seventy patients were examined at baseline and again, after 3 and after 6 months of antipsychotic medication. Sexual dysfunction and loss of libido were not rated using a specific rating scale. The sample was divided into three groups: olanzapine, risperidone and first-generation antipsychotics. At baseline, prior to taking any medication, 37% of the patients reported some sexual dysfunctions. After being treated, patients receiving olanzapine showed the lowest rate of loss of libido and of sexual dysfunction. These findings are in line with an older, double-blind study that compared olanzapine to risperidone in the treatment of schizophrenia patients [27]. Sexual dysfunction was significantly lower in olanzapine-treated patients than in those treated with risperidone.

A large sample of 3,828 schizophrenia outpatients was examined by Dossenbach et al. [28]. The outpatients were treated with either olanzapine (n = 2,638), risperidone (n = 860), quetiapine (n = 142) or haloperidol (n = 188). Sexual dysfunction was evaluated through patients' and investigators' perception using the UKU Side Effect Rating Scale. Patients in the olanzapine-treated and quetiapine-treated groups experienced significantly less sexual dysfunction (55.7 and 60.2%, respectively) than patients who received risperidone (67.8%) or haloperidol (71.1%). Quetiapine and ziprasidone have not been associated with elevated prolactin levels [21, 29]. The lower propensity of quetiapine to cause sexual dysfunction has also been demonstrated in several recent studies [30]. Controlled studies for sexual dysfunction induced by ziprasidone are still needed.

In recent years, reports about the efficacy of treatment with sildenafil (Viagra) in sexual disorders in schizophrenia patients have been accumulating. Case reports and an open-label study, as well as clinical experience of psychiatrists revealed that sildenafil may be an efficient treatment in less deteriorated patients who are capable of having a proper relationship with their spouse [31, 32].

This has also been demonstrated in a double-blind placebo-controlled study [33]. Thirty-two patients with ED suffering from schizophrenia or delusional disorder randomly received either sildenafil (25 mg, 1–2 times per day) or placebo, and were crossed over to the other arm after 2 weeks. Duration and frequency of erections, as well as satisfaction with intercourse, were superior in sildenafil-treated patients. The drug was well tolerated; therefore, the authors suggest that sildenafil can be a useful approach in treating ED in schizophrenia patients.

In summary, the therapeutic approach to sexual dysfunction in schizophrenia patients should be according to the following stages: (1) adjusting medication to minimal effective dose; (2) switching to atypical antipsychotics: quetiapine, olanzapine, ziprazidone or clozapine; (3) psychotherapy: couple/family intervention to restore relationship; (4) in males, addition of a PDE-5 inhibitor (sildenafil, vardenafil, tadalafil).

Sexual Dysfunction in Patients Suffering from Depression

About 10% of the population suffers from depressive episodes with a severe impairment in the quality of life and functioning. Decreased libido commonly accompanies an episode of major depression. Casper et al. [34], in the classic study on a sample of moderate to severe hospitalized drug-free patients with major affective disorder, found that the majority of these patients (72% of unipolar depressed, 77% of bipolar depressed) experienced loss of sexual interest. Increasing severity of depression and anxiety were associated with loss of libido. Age and cognitive impairment also showed a strong correlation with the reduction in sexual interest. Depressed patients with increased appetite were more sensitive in personal relationships, more hostile and reported a greater decrease in libido than the matched depressed group without increased appetite. Depressed persons may also experience diminished ability to maintain sexual arousal or achieve orgasm. In males with severe depression, the rate of ED might reach 90% [35]. Assessment of nocturnal penile tumescence has been used as a measure of erectile capacity. Thase et al. [36] studied a sample of 34 male outpatients with major depression and an age-matched group of 28 healthy controls. Diminution of penile rigidity was found in approximately 40% of the depressed outpatients in addition to a reduction in the duration (in minutes) of sleep-related tumescence (nocturnal penile tumescence time) when compared to the healthy controls [37]. These findings were replicated in a second sample of 51 depressed male outpatients [37]. Thus, it seems that depression in men is associated with a potentially reversible decrease in erectile capacity which may be associated with significant sexual dysfunction.

Depression is widely treated with antidepressants. The treatment is usually prolonged, for a period of months to years and demands cooperation from the patient. Selective serotonin reuptake inhibitors (SSRIs) replaced gradually tricyclic antidepressants (TCAs). SSRIs have less side effects than TCAs, mainly due to lack of the anticholinergic side effects. However, one of the salient side effects of SSRIs is impairment of sexual function. The most prominent effect is inhibition of orgasm, but also impairment in desire and arousal, and as a consequence the feeling of satisfaction from sexual function is negatively affected [3].

The evaluation of the prevalence of sexual dysfunction as a result of medical treatment is not simple, as the depressive state itself may affect sexual desire and arousal. Significant differences in prevalence may be found according to the assessment methodology used. Early studies were based on standard registration of side effects. Later studies are based on patients' responses to specific questioning on sexual side effects or on structured questionnaires. Many patients did not report spontaneously on their sexual dysfunction since they did not relate it to medication or did not think that their dysfunction is of interest to the treating physician. A good evaluation of a dysfunction should therefore rely on a structured questionnaire which intentionally inquires the change in each of the components of the sexual cycle, namely, desire, arousal and orgasm in comparison to the state before initiation of medical treatment and the basic state of that person.

A high incidence of sexual dysfunction has previously been reported with the TCAs and the monoamine oxidase inhibitors. In a controlled study from 1986 on a heterogeneous population of males and females, Harrison et al. [38] found that 30% of depressed patients treated with the TCA imipramine and 40% of patients treated with the monoamine oxidase inhibitor phenelzine complained on sexual dysfunction compared to a rate of 6% on placebo. A double-blind study in obsessive-compulsive patients treated with clomipramine 100–150 mg/day, found an orgasmic impairment in 23 out of 24 patients (96%) [39]. When the first SSRI fluoxetine was introduced, the 45th edition of Physicians' Desk Reference reported an incidence of sexual dysfunction of 1.9% for men and women combined [40]. Controlled studies confirmed the clinical impression that the incidence of sexual dysfunction is much higher and reaches up to 75% for delayed orgasm in patients treated with fluoxetine [41]. The rates of sexual dysfunction reported with SSRIs range from 34 to 78% of patients across studies in which patients were questioned directly about their sexual functioning [4, 5, 42–43].

A recent study estimated the prevalence of antidepressant-induced sexual dysfunction in a cross-sectional survey of 502 adults in France and the UK [44]. The prevalence was obtained from the patients' responses to the question regarding changes in sexual functioning since the initiation of SSRIs or serotonin-norepinephrine reuptake inhibitors (SNRIs). Using this definition of antidepressant-induced sexual dysfunction attributable to SSRI or SNRI treatment, the estimated prevalence of sexual dysfunction was 39.2% for the UK sample and 26.6% for the French sample.

Similarly, the prevalence of sexual dysfunction in a large US clinical sample based on the changes in sexual functioning questionnaire [45] was 37% for all antidepressants combined and ranged from 22 to 43% across antidepressants [4]. In this study, SSRIs (citalopram, sertraline, paroxetine and fluoxetine) and the SNRI venlafaxine were associated with high incidence of sexual dysfunction. The highest rates were in the paroxetine group (43%). The lowest rates were for the bupropion (22%) and the nefazodone (28%) groups. Some studies [43, 46] have found that paroxetine provoked significantly more delay in orgasm or ejaculation and more frequent ED than fluvoxamine, fluoxetine and sertraline. In a more recent study by Landen et al. [47] no statistically significant difference regarding incidence of sexual dysfunction, was found between citalopram and paroxetine. The high incidence of sexual dysfunctions with SSRIs and SNRIs suggests that the common mechanism of action involves activation of the 5-HT2 receptor. An explanation for the apparently greater incidence of sexual dysfunction in patients receiving paroxetine may be related to the affinity of paroxetine to the cholinergic receptor [3]. Bupropion, a norepinephrine-dopamine reuptake inhibitor, does not have a direct effect on serotonin. These properties may explain the low incidence of sexual dysfunction associated with this antidepressant [48].

The incidence of treatment-emergent sexual dysfunction of duloxetine, a newer SNRI, was assessed in four double-blind paroxetine and placebo-controlled trials [49] in patients with major depression. The incidence was significantly lower in patients treated with duloxetine than in patients treated with paroxetine, although both rates were higher than observed in patients taking placebo.

The antidepressants from the SSRIs group are devoid of significant activity on the adrenergic, cholinergic and histaminergic receptors, thus the mechanism of the sexual dysfunction caused by these medications is probably related to the activation of the serotonergic system. Studies on animals showed, indeed, that increased central serotonergic activity inhibits sexual behavior. The 5-HT2 receptors have an important role in this activity. The dopaminergic system, on the other hand, increases sexual behavior, mainly arousal [9].

The therapeutic approaches to sexual dysfunction induced by SSRIs are all based on attenuation of the central serotonergic activity or stimulation of the dopaminergic activity. In patients that are not troubled by their sexual dysfunction, it is possible to wait several weeks, and sometimes the side effects can be resolved spontaneously. When it is clinically possible, the dose of the medication may be reduced. Another form of decreasing the dose is to halt medication for a day or two before planned sexual relationship (drug holiday) [50]. This approach can be effective only with medication with a short half-life time like paroxetine or sertraline but not with fluoxetine, which has a long half-life time. The disadvantage of drug holidays is the need to plan the sexual life.

Cyproheptadine, an antihistaminergic agent with antagonistic activity at the 5-HT2 receptors was found effective, as adjunct to SSRIs, in restoration of sexual function. It is administered in a dose of 4–12 mg, an hour or two before sexual relationship. However, in some patients it caused marked sedation [51]. Coadministration of mianserin, an antidepressant with 5-HT2a/2c and α_2-antagonistic activity, was studied in men and women with sexual dysfunction due to SSRIs [52, 53]. Nine out of 15 men and 10 out of 16 women showed marked improvement mainly in orgasm and satisfaction from sexual relationships. The dose was 15 mg/day and the improvement in sexual function was achieved within 2 weeks. Nefazodone combines in its mechanism of action serotonin reuptake inhibitory reactivity with antagonistic activity at the 5-HT2 receptors. In a double-blind study, patients treated with nefazodone showed indeed significantly less sexual dysfunction compared to sertraline [54].

An additional strategy, via the serotonergic system, is the addition of the antianxiety drug buspirone. In a retrospective, open trial, 11 of 16 patients showed improvement in sexual desire and in orgasm disorder, with a dose of 15–60 mg per day [55]. This observation was confirmed in a double-blind, placebo-controlled study of 117 assessable patients. Landén et al. [56] demonstrated that the addition of buspirone (20–60 mg/day) to SSRI therapy for 4 weeks led to remission of sexual dysfunction (decreased desire and/or impaired orgasm) in 58% of patients, compared with 30% of placebo controls. The differences were significant starting in the 2nd week. The presumed mechanism is reduction in serotonergic activity by the activation of the 5-HT1a receptor. It is not clear if buspirone is effective for cases of ED as well. However, another study failed to demonstrate a beneficial effect of buspirone add-on in female depressed patients [57].

Another treatment approach is to enhance dopaminergic activity. A number of successful cases resulting from the addition of the dopaminergic drugs amantadine (100–200 mg per day), dextroamphetamine, methylphenidate (Ritalin) and pemoline, were reported [3].

When appropriate clinically, switching to alternative medication should be considered. Such alternatives include: bupropion, mirtazapine and reboxetine. Several studies demonstrated that replacing the SSRI treatment with bupropion, or sustained-release bupropion, resulted in disappearance of the sexual dysfunction in most patients [48, 58]. Bupropion has been shown to be effective also when used as an antidote to SSRIs [59]. The antidepressant mirtazapine as well, is associated with less propensity to cause sexual dysfunction, as compared to SSRIs, a property which can be attributed to its antagonistic activity at the 5-HT2 and the α_2-receptors [60]. Switching to the selective norepinephrine reuptake inhibitor reboxetine may be another option for patients with SSRI-induced sexual dysfunctions [61].

The addition of sildenafil to patients treated with antidepressant-induced sexual dysfunction was found to be effective. Nurnberg [62] found that the effectiveness of sildenafil in 65 patients who were also being treated with antidepressants was not different from its effectiveness in 2,050 men without SSRIs. This has been confirmed in later randomized controlled studies [63]. Sildenafil given in a flexible dose was well tolerated and significantly improved erectile function, arousal, ejaculation, orgasm and overall sexual satisfaction in men with ED associated with SSRI therapy for depression. Sildenafil (25–50 mg/day) appeared to reverse ED also in 8 out of 11 elderly depressed male patients (mean age 73 years) treated with SSRIs [64].

In conclusion, patients treated with SSRIs have a high incidence of sexual dysfunction. This results in serious deterioration of the quality of life and causes the patients to stop drug treatment. Addition of medications that block serotonergic activity in the 5-HT2 receptor help some patients resolve the problems and reach orgasm. When clinically appropriate, it is advisable to switch to medications that cause less sexual dysfunction (bupropion, mirtazapine, nefazodone, reboxetine). ED caused by affective disorders or by treatment with SSRIs can be improved significantly with sildenafil and probably also with its two compatible drugs tadalafil and vardenafil.

Anxiety Disorders and Sexual Functioning

Anxiety is an important factor in the development of sexual dysfunctions [6, 65]. The phenomenon of performance anxiety is well known, particularly in men who are concerned over their erectile response and durability of the erection. Narcissistic perturbation is yet another psychological consequence of ED that further increases anxiety. The patient's self-esteem may sink further causing concern for both himself and his partner. This may result in behavioral modifications in the patient, such as avoiding intimacy and temper outbursts. These lead to increasing anxiety and increasing ED resulting in a vicious cycle of failure and escalating anxiety. This specific situation can be treated in most cases with the help of explanations and short-term therapeutic intervention intended to relieve anxiety.

Roughly 15% of the population suffers from various kinds of anxiety disorders. Those include generalized anxiety disorder, panic disorder, obsessive-compulsive disorder (OCD), social phobia (SP) and posttraumatic stress disorder (PTSD).

Research, dating back to the 80s, shows that people with high levels of anxiety have a higher rate of sexual dysfunctions [6]. Although the psychoanalytic literature has directed much attention to the association of anxiety provoked by intrapsychiatric conflicts and sexual dysfunction [66], there is little information on the comorbidity of sexual dysfunction and anxiety disorders. Kaplan [6] claimed that the role of anxiety is especially clear in the pathogenesis of sexual aversion disorders and phobic avoidance of sex. She found an unexpectedly high incidence of panic disorders in patients who phobically avoid sex or who complain of active sexual aversion. Some of the patients actually experienced panic about their sexual performance or became obsessed with details concerning their sexual performance and loss of control. Monteiro et al. [39] found a high percentage of sexual pathology in untreated patients with OCD of whom up to 24% were virgins and another 9% had not had sex for years.

SP and Sexual Behavior

The main component of SP is extreme fear of public behavior that may cause embarrassment or ridicule. This is a combination of performance anxiety and interpersonal anxiety that exists in 7% of the population. It is reasonable to expect that this type of anxiety disorder is accompanied by sexual dysfunction.

Heimberg and Barlow [67] hypothesized that sexual dysfunction (especially reduced erectile capability) is a result of performance anxiety or fear of scrutiny by others, similar to SP. Using a laboratory model, they found that healthy men exposed to both erotic stimuli and anxiety-provoking stimuli showed increased arousal compared to healthy men exposed to erotic stimuli alone. However, in sexually dysfunctional males, the opposite occurred: they reacted to the anxiety-provoking stimuli with decreased arousal. The authors concluded that anxiety apparently affects sexually functional and dysfunctional males in opposite ways and that dysfunctional males may employ the same cognitive model as patients with SP.

There are several studies suggesting that patients with SP may have sexual problems. In a study of college students, Leary and Dobbins [68] reported that subjects with a high rate of 'heterosocial anxiety' showed a higher incidence of sexual dysfunction. Figueira et al. [69] reported a 33.3% rate of sexual difficulties, especially premature ejaculation, in patients with SP.

Bodinger et al. [70] evaluated 40 consecutive, drug-free outpatients with SP (24 males, 16 females) attending an anxiety clinic, and 40 healthy, age and gender-matched controls. A detailed rating scale was used to assess quantitatively and qualitatively sexual function and behavior [71]. The findings showed that men suffering from SP reported moderate impairment in sexual enjoyment and subjective sexual satisfaction. In addition, the men reported a later age for first sexual experience and a higher rate (42%) of paid for sex as compared to the healthy men (8%). Women suffering from SP reported severe impairment in desire, arousal, sexual activity and subjective satisfaction. These women had less sexual partners compared to the healthy controls. Seven out of 16 (44%) had only one partner or none throughout their lifetime, compared with 6% in the control group. Both men and women showed avoidance of intergender behavior.

PTSD and Sexual Disorders

Exposure to extreme traumatic events (military, traffic accident, rape) may lead to behavioral and physiological abnormalities which at times persist long after the precipitating event and become permanent, leading to the clinical syndrome known as PTSD. PTSD is known to affect significantly emotional, social, occupational and sexual functioning. Kaplan [6, 72] has shown that sexual problems are prevalent among PTSD patients. Letourneau et al. [7] reported that over 80% of PTSD patients studied, were experiencing clinically relevant difficulties. ED and premature ejaculation were the most frequently reported problems. They suggest that PTSD may be a risk factor for sexual problems [7]. PTSD patients are frequently treated for symptoms of anxiety and depression, mainly with anxiolytics and antidepressants. Fossey and Hamner

[73] reported that clonazepam can cause sexual dysfunction in male veterans with PTSD. The role of antidepressants in inducing sexual dysfunction is well known [3].

A study by Kotler et al. [74] compared the various components of sexual functioning among three groups of males: untreated PTSD patients (n = 15), PTSD patients being treated with SSRIs (n = 27) and a group of healthy controls (n = 49). All participants completed an 18-item questionnaire for assessment of sexual functioning [71]. Those with PTSD also completed the impact of events scale [75] and the symptom checklist-90 [76]. Untreated and treated PTSD patients had significantly poorer sexual functioning in all domains (desire, arousal, orgasm, activity and satisfaction). Compared to healthy controls, those treated with SSRIs had greater impairment in desire, arousal and frequency of sexual activity with a partner. There was a high correlation between sexual dysfunction among the PTSD group and the anger-hostility subscale of the symptom checklist-90.

Treating male PTSD sufferers with sildenafil in a dose of 50 mg brought about significant improvement (53.5%) in erection functionality and at the same time improved desire, orgasm and sexual satisfaction [77]. This study shows that the phases of the sexual cycle are connected to each other and improving one usually results in improvement of the other phases.

In conclusion, anxiety disorders are associated with a significant impairment in all domains of sexual functioning.

Sexual Dysfunction in Patients with Eating Disorders

Clinicians have often reported that anorexia nervosa (AN) patients suffer from sexual dysfunction and immaturity, as manifested in low sexual interest, inhibited sexual behavior, disgust towards sex and fear of intimacy [78–82]. This can be expected since persons with AN are characterized by a profound disturbance of body image and feel overweight or misshapen. AN is much more prevalent in females than in males and its onset is usually in adolescence. Most research on eating disorders and sexuality has been done on women.

Raboch and Faltus [79] investigated the sexual development and sexual function of 30 adult women with AN and of 50 control women using a structured interview and 3 sexological self-report questionnaires. The average age of patients and controls was 24 years. Nineteen of the 30 patients (63%) had irregular menstruation or secondary amenorrhea. They were mostly unmarried and often without a satisfactory partner relationship. At examination time, 20% of the patients had no coital experience and 80% were found to have sexual disturbances. In comparison, 92% of the control group reported having a satisfactory partner relationship.

This study and others [78, 81] have shown that during adolescence, prior to becoming anorectic, the sexual development of AN patients was normal [81] or even accelerated [78]. During their anorectic period, patients reported a considerable decrease in sexual interest and need for intimacy [81]. Biological and psychological factors may contribute to this unfavorable state.

Morgan [82] studied the sexual functioning and attitudes of 57 former eating disorder, female patients who had received treatment 2 years or more prior to the reported evaluation. Of this group of 31 AN (i.e. restricting) patients and 26 bulimia (i.e. purging) patients, 42 returned the self-report questionnaire. Participants ranged in age from 18 to 42 years. The large majority of respondents (85.7%) were married, engaged or involved in an exclusive dating relationship. Former anorectic patients were less likely to return the questionnaire. Among those who returned it, formerly anorectic women were less likely to be in a romantic/erotic relationship and were significantly less likely to have engaged in masturbation than former bulimics and also scored lower on a measure of sexual esteem. No differences were found between the two groups with regard to frequency of orgasm or intercourse. When both eating disorder groups were compared with a normative sample, the eating disorder patients reported decreased frequency of masturbation and intercourse, lower orgasmic responsiveness and more negative affect during sex. Nearly 40% of the eating disorder patients reported clinically significant levels of sexual discord with their current partner.

One may conclude that eating disorder patients, even after recovery, struggle with acceptance of their sexuality and have high rates of inhibited sexual desire, sexual aversion and anorgasmia. The psychosexual therapy of patients with eating disorders is complicated due to basic issues of control, grounded in these patients' early lives and intense resistance to psychotherapy [80]. Eating disorder patients exhibit problematic personality characteristics, with a high frequency of secondary diagnoses of borderline or narcissistic personality disorders as well as depressive states. The general treatment approach is to educate these patients as much as possible about sexuality and desensitize them to their own body [80].

Sexual Dysfunction in Patients with Personality Disorders

Patients with personality disorders show deeply ingrained, inflexible and maladaptive patterns of relating to and perceiving both the environment and themselves. The relational style of people with borderline personality disorder (BPD) is characterized in the DSM-IV criteria as intense and unstable, marked further by abandonment fears and by vacillating between idealization and devaluation. Additional criteria are identity disturbance, impulsivity and inappropriate intense anger. It seems reasonable to expect that these disturbed relationship traits may interfere with sexual functioning and the capacity for intimacy.

There are, however, very few studies that address specifically the sexual relationships of patients with personality disorders. A 1986 study [78] examined 30 women, of an average age of 34 years, hospitalized for decompensation of ICD-9 'hysterical psychopathic personality'. Using questionnaires designed specifically for the assessment of sexual development, it was found that these patients displayed disharmonious sexual development. On other questionnaires, they exhibited lower scores on sexual function, decreased sexual activity and a lower coital orgasmic capacity [78].

A more recent study examined a large (n = 290) and well-defined sample of BPD patients and 72 Axis II non-borderline comparison subjects, followed prospectively for 6 years. Sexual relationship difficulties were common among BPD patients and significantly more common among them than in the Axis II comparison group. Sixty-one percent of BPD patients reported some type of sexual relationship difficulty versus 19% of other personality disorder patients. Within the BPD group, these difficulties were more common among women. Sixty-five percent of female BPD and 43% of male BPD patients reported either becoming symptomatic (e.g. becoming dissociated, feeling suicidal, hurting self) as a result of having consenting sex, or avoiding sex for fear of suffering from symptoms, or both. These behavioral patterns decline significantly with time. Notably, a higher percentage of BPD patients with a history of sexual relationship difficulties had reported a childhood history of sexual abuse (76.8%) compared to BPD patients without such history (39.8%). Much the same pattern was found in patients with an adult history of rape (42.9 vs. 13.3%).

The authors suggest that the sexual trauma, which is so common in BPD patients, whether in childhood, adulthood or both, would predispose many of these people to avoidance of sexual experiences for fear of triggering a recrudescence of trauma-related memories, BPD symptoms, or both. The between-gender differential rates of childhood sexual abuse and adult rape histories reported in this study [83] help to explain the difference in rates of sexual relationship difficulties between male and female BPD patients.

The sexual difficulties of BPD patients stem from the recurrent interpersonal problems they experience with family members, intimate partners, and other significant persons in their lives. It is possible that addressing adequately the fears of these patients may help improve the quality of their interpersonal adult relationships, including sexual relationships.

Conclusions

The rate of sexual dysfunction in patients suffering from psychiatric disorders like schizophrenia, depression, anxiety disorders, eating disorders and personality disorders is significantly high. The psychotropic medications used for treating these disorders often exacerbate the sexual dysfunction. For the patient who clearly suffers from sexual dysfunction, it is not sufficient to label it a psychogenic reason. Rather, it is necessary to diagnose the problems and treat them specifically. It seems that the new drugs from the 5-phosphodiesterase inhibitor group (sildenafil, tadalafil, vardenafil) have the potential to overcome the specific psychiatric or physical problem providing a personal relationship that is satisfying and devoid of anger and hostility.

References

1 Laumann EO, Paik A, Rosen RC: Sexual dysfunction in the United States prevalence and predictors. JAMA 1999;281:537–544.

2 Peuskens J, Sienaert P, De Hert M: Sexual dysfunction: the unspoken side effect of antipsychotics. Eur Psychiatry 1998;13:23s–30s.

3 Rosen RC, Lane RM, Menza M: Effects of SSRI's on sexual function: a critical review. J Clin Psychopharmacol 1999;19:67–85.

4 Clayton AH, Pradko JF, Croft HA, Montano CB, Leadbetter RA, Bolden-Watson C, Bass KI, Donahue RMJ, Jamerson BD, Metz A: Prevalence of sexual dysfunction among newer antidepressants. J Clin Psychiatry 2002;63:357–366.

5 Osvath P, Fekete S, Voros V, Vitrai J: Sexual dysfunction among patients treated with antidepressants – a Hungarian retrospective study. Eur Psychiatry 2003; 18:412–414.

6 Kaplan HS: Anxiety and sexual dysfunction. J Clin Psychiatry 1988;49:21–25.

7 Letourneau EJ, Schewe PA, Frueh BC: Preliminary evaluation of sexual problems in combat veterans with PTSD. J Trauma Stress 1997;10:125–132.

8 Pfaus JG, Everitt BJ: The psychopharmacology of sexual behavior; in Bloom FE, Kupfer DJ (eds): Psychopharmacology: The Fourth Generation of Progress. New York, Raven Press, 1995, pp 743–758.

9 Meston CM, Frohlich PF: The neurobiology of sexual function. Arch Gen Psychiatry 2000;57:1012–1030.

10 Finkel MS, Laghrissi-Thode F, Pollock BG, Rong J: Paroxetine is a novel nitric oxide sythase inhibitor. Psychopharmacol Bull 1996;32:653–658.

11 Kotin J, Wibert DE, Verburg D, Soldinger SM: Thioridazine and sexual dysfunction. Am J Psychiatry 1976;133:82–85.

12 Ghadirian AM, Chouinard G, Annable L. Sexual dysfunction and plasma prolactin levels in neuroleptic-treated schizophrenic outpatients. J Nerv Ment Dis 1982;170:463–467.

13 Smith SM, O'Keane V, Murray R: Sexual dysfunction in patients taking conventional antipsychotic medication. Br J Psychiatry 2002;181:49–55.

14 Aizenberg D, Zemishlany Z, Dorfman-Etrog P, Weizman A: Sexual dysfunction in male schizophrenic patients. J Clin Psychiatry 1995;56:137–141.

15 Macdonald S, Halliday J, MacEwan T, Sharkey V, Farrington S, Wall S, McCreadie RG: Nithsdale schizophrenia surveys 24: sexual dysfunction. Br J Psychiatry 2003;182:50–56.

16 Angrist B, Gershon S: Clinical response to several dopamine agonists of schizophrenic and non-schizophrenic subjects. Adv Biochem Psychopharmacol 1977;16:677–680.

17 Schiavi RC, Segraves RT: The biology of sexual function. Psychiatr Clin North Am 1995;18:7–23.

18 Valevski A, Modai I, Zbarski E, Zemishlany Z, Weizman A: Effect of amantadine on sexual dysfunction in neuroleptic-treated male schizophrenic patients. Clin Neuropharmacol 1998;21:355–357.

19 Berry MD, Juorio AV, Pasteron IA: Possible mechanisms of action of deprenyl and other MAO-B inhibitors in some neurologic and psychiatric disorders. Prog Neurobiol 1994;44:141–161.

20 Kodesh A, Weizman A, Aizenberg D, Hermesh H, Gelkopf M, Zemishlany Z: Selegiline in the treatment of sexual dysfunction in schizophrenia patients maintained on neuroleptics: a pilot study. Clin Neuropharmacol 2003;26:193–195.

21 Cutler AJ: Sexual dysfunction and antipsychotic treatment. Psychoneuroendocrinology 2003;28:69–82.

22 Hummer M, Kemmler G, Kurz M, Kurzthaler I, Oberbauer H, Fleischhacker W: Sexual disturbances during clozapine and haloperidol treatment for schizophrenia. Am J Psychiatry 1999;156:631–633.

23 Aizenberg D, Modai I, Landa A, Gil-Ad I, Weizman A: Comparison of sexual dysfunction in male schizophrenic patients maintained on treatment with classical antipsychotics versus clozapine. J Clin Psychiatry 2001;62:541–544.

24 Kleinberg DK, Davis JM, de Coster R, Van Baelen B, Brecher M: Prolactin levels and adverse events in patients treated with resperidone. J Clin Psychopharmacol 1999;19:57–61.

25 Peuskens J: Risperidone in the treatment of patients with chronic schizophrenia: a multinational, multicentre, double-blind, parallel group study versus haloperidol. Br J Psychiatry 1995;166:712–726.

26 Bitter I, Basson BR, Dossenbach MR: Antipsychotic treatment and sexual functioning in first-time neuroleptic-treated schizophrenic patients. Int Chil Psychopharmacol 2005;20:19–21.

27 Tran PV, Hamilton SH, Kuntz AJ, Potvin JH, Andersen SW, Beasley C, Tollefson GD: Double-blind comparison of olanzapine versus risperidone in the treatment of schizophrenia and other psychotic disorders. J Clin Psychopharmacol 1997;17:407–418.

28 Dossenbach M, Dyachkova Y, Pirildar S, Anders M, Khalil A, Araszkiewicz A, Shakhnovich T, Akram A, Pecenak J, McBride M, Treuer T: Effects of atypical and typical antipsychotic treatments on sexual function in patients with schizophrenia: 12-month results from the Intercontinental Schizophrenia Outpatient Health Outcomes (IC-SOHO) study. Eur Psychiatry 2006;21:251–258.

29 Hamner M: The effect of atypical antipsychotics on serum prolactin levels. Ann Clin Psychiatry 2002; 14:163–173.

30 Kelly DL, Conley RR: A randomized double-blind 12 week study of quetiapine, risperidone or fluphenazine on sexual functioning in people with schizophrenia. Psychoneuroendocrinology 2006;31:340–346.
31 Benatov R, Reznik I, Zemishlany Z: Sildenafil citrate (Viagra) treatment of sexual dysfunction in a schizophrenic patient. Eur Psychiatry 1999;14: 353–355.
32 Aviv A, Shelef A, Weizman A: An open-label trial of sildenafil addition in risperidone-treated male schizophrenia patients with erectile dysfunction. J Clin Psychiatry 2004;65:97–103.
33 Gopalakrishnan R, Jacob KS, Kuruvilla A, Vasantharaj B, John JK: Sildenafil in the treatment of antipsychotic-induced erectile dysfunction: a randomized, double-blind, placebo-controlled, flexible-dose, two-way crossover trial. Am J Psychiatry 2006; 163:494–499.
34 Casper RC, Redmond DE, Katz MM, Schaffer CB, Davis JM, Doslow SH: Somatic symptoms in primary affective disorder. Arch Gen Psychiatry 1985; 42:1098–1104.
35 Feldman HA, Goldstein I, Hatzichristou DG, Krane RJ, McKinlay JB: Impotence and its medical and psychosocial correlates: results of the Massachusetts Male Aging Study. J Urol 1994;151:54–61.
36 Thase ME, Reynolds CF III, Jennings JR, Frank E, Howell JR, Houck PR, Berman S, Kupfer D: Nocturnal penile tumexcence is diminished in depressed men. Biol Psychiatry 1988;24:33–46.
37 Thase ME, Reynolds CF III, Jennings JR, Frank E, Garamoni GL, Nofzinger EA, Fascizka AL, Kupfer DJ: Diminished nocturnal penile tumescence in depression: a repliaction study. Biol Psychiatry 1992; 31:1136–1142.
38 Harrison WM, Rabkin JG, Ehrhardt AA, Stewart JW, McGrath PJ, Ross D, Quitkin FM: Effects of antidepressant medication on sexual function: a controlled study. J Clin Psychopharmacol 1986;6:144–149.
39 Monteiro WO, Noshirvani HF, Marks IM, Lelliott PT: Anorgasmia from clomipramine in obsessive-compulsive disorder: a controlled trial. Br J Psychiatry 1987;151:107–112.
40 Physicians' desk reference, ed 45. Oradell NJ, Medical Economics Data, 1991, p 904.
41 Patterson WM: Fluoxetine-induced sexual dysfunction. J Clin Psychiatry 1993;54:71.
42 Balon R, Yeragani VK, Pohl R, Ramesh C: Sexual dysfunction during antidepressant treatment. J Clin Psychiatry 1993;54:209–212.
43 Montejo-González AL, Llorca G, Izquierdo JA, Ledesma A, Bousoño M, Calcedo A, Carrasco JL, Ciudad J, Daniel E, De la Gandara J, Derecho J, Franco M, Gomez MJ, Macias JA, Martin T, Perez V, Sanchez JM, Sanchez S, Vicens E: SSRI-induced sexual dysfunction: fluoxetine, paroxetine, sertraline, and fluvoxamine in a prospective, multicenter, and descriptive clinical study of 344 patients. J Sex Marital Ther 1997;23:176–194.
44 Williams VS, Baldwin DS, Hogue SL, Fehnel SE, Hollis KA, Edin HM: Estimating the prevalence and impact of antidepressant-induced sexual dysfunction in 2 European countries: a cross-sectional patient survey. J Clin Psychiatry 2006;67:204–210.
45 Clayton AH, McGarvey EL, Clavet GJ: The Changes in Sexual Functioning Questionnaire (CSFQ): development, reliability, and validity. Psychopharmacol Bull 1997;33:731–745.
46 Waldinger MD, Hengeveld MW, Zwinderman AH, Olivier B: Effect of SSRI antidepressants on ejaculation: a double-blind, randomized, placebo-controlled study with fluoxetine, fluvoxamine, paroxetine, and sertraline. J Clin Psychopharmacol 1998;18:274–281.
47 Landén M, Högberg P, Thase ME: Incidence of sexual side effects in refractory depression during treatment with citalopram or paroxetine. J Clin Psychiatry 2005;66:100–106.
48 Walker PW, Cole JO, Gardner EA, Hughes AR, Johnston JA, Batey SR, Lineberry CG: Improvement in fluoxetine-associated sexual dysfunction in patients switched to bupropion. J Clin Psychiatry 1993;54:459–465.
49 Delgado PL, Brannan SK, Mallinckrodt CH, Tran PV, McNamara RK, Wang F, Watkin JG, Detke MJ: Sexual functioning assessed in 4 double-blind placebo- and paroxetine-controlled trials of duloxetine for major depressive disorder. J Clin Psychiatry 2005;66:686–692.
50 Rothschild AJ: Selective serotonin reuptake inhibitor-induced sexual dysfunction: efficacy of a drug holiday. Am J Psychiatry 1995;152:1514–1516.
51 Aizenberg D, Zemishlany Z, Weizman A: Cyproheptadine treatment of sexual dysfunction induced by serotonin reuptake inhibitors. Clin Neuropharmacol 1995;18:320–324.
52 Aizenberg D, Gur S, Zemishlany Z, Granek M, Jeczmien P, Weizman A: Mianserin, a 5-HT2a/2c and alpha 2 antagonist, in the treatment of sexual dysfunction induced by serotonin reuptake inhibitors. Clin Neuropharmacol 1997;20:210–214.
53 Aizenberg D, Naor S, Zemishlany Z, Weizman A: The serotonin antagonist mianserin for treatment of serotonin reuptake inhibitor-induced sexual dysfunction in women: an open-label add-on study. Clin Neuropharmacol 1999;22:347–350.

54 Feiger A, Kiev A, Shrivastava RK, Wisselink PG, Wilcox CS: Nefazodone versus sertraline in outpatients with major depression: focus on efficacy, tolerability, and effects on sexual function and satisfaction. J Clin Psychiatry 1996;57:53–62.
55 Norden MJ: Buspirone treatement of sexual dysfunction associated with selective serotonin reuptake inhibitors. Depression 1994;2:109–112.
56 Landén M, Eriksson E, Agren H, Fahlén T: Effect of buspirone on sexual dysfunction in depressed patients treated with selective serotonin reuptake inhibitors. J Clin Psychopharmacol 1999;19:268–271.
57 Michelson D, Bancroft J, Targum S, Kim Y, Tepner R: Female sexual dysfunction associated with antidepressant administration: a randomized, placebo-controlled study of pharmacologic intervention. Am J Psychiatry 2000;157:239–243.
58 Masand PS, Ashton AK, Gupta S, Frank B: Sustained-release bupropion for selective serotonin reuptake inhibitor-induced sexual dysfunction: a randomized, double-blind, placebo-controlled, parallel-group study. Am J Psychiatry 2001;158:805–807.
59 Clayton AH, Warnock JK, Kornstein SG, Pinkerton R, Sheldon-Keller A, McGarvey EL: A placebo-controlled trial of bupropion SR as an antidote for selective serotonin reuptake inhibitor-induced sexual dysfunction. J Clin Psychiatry 2004;65:62–67.
60 Koutouvidis N, Pratikakis M, Fotiadou A: The use of mirtazapine in a group of 11 patients following poor compliance to selective serotonin reuptake inhibitor treatment due to sexual dysfunction. Int Clin Psychopharmacol 1999;14:253–255.
61 Clayton AH, Zajecka J, Ferguson JM, Filipiak-Reisner JK, Brown MT, Schwartz GE: Lack of sexual dysfunction with the selective noradrenaline reuptake inhibitor reboxetine during treatment for major depressive disorder. Int Clin Psychopharmacol 2003;18:151–156.
62 Nurnberg HG, Gelenberg A, Hargreave TB, Harrison WM, Siegel RL, Smith MD: Efficacy of sildenafil citrate for the treatment of erectile dysfunction in men taking serotonin reuptake inhibitors. Am J Psychiatry 2001;158:1926–1928.
63 Fava M, Nurnberg HG, Seidman SN, Holloway W, Nicholas S, Tseng LJ, Stecher VJ: Efficacy and safety of sildenafil in men with serotonergic antidepressant-associated erectile dysfunction: results from a randomized, double-blind, placebo-controlled trial. J Clin Psychiatry 2006;67:240–246.
64 Aizenberg D, Weizman A, Barak Y: Sildenafil for selective serotonin reuptake inhibitor-induced erectile dysfunction in elderly male depressed patients. J Sex Marital Ther 2003;29:297–303.
65 Hedon F: Anxiety and erectile dysfunction: a global approach to ED enhances results and quality of life. Int J Impot Res 2003;15:S16–S19.
66 Janssen PL: Psychodynamic study of male potency disorders. An overview. Psychother Psychosom 1985;44:6–17.
67 Heimberg RG, Barlow DH: Psychosocial treatments for social phobia. Psychosomatics 1988;29:27–37.
68 Leary MR, Dobbins SE: Social anxiety, sexual behavior, and contraceptive use. J Pers Soc Psychol 1983;45:1347–1354.
69 Figueira I, Possidente E, Marques C, Hayes K: Sexual dysfunction: a neglected complication of panic disorder and social phobia. Arch Sex Behav 2001; 30:369–377.
70 Bodinger L, Hermesh H, Aizenberg D, Valevski A, Marom S, Shiloh R, Gothelf D, Zemishlany Z, Weizman A: Sexual function and behavior in social phobia. J Clin Psychiatry 2002;63:874–879.
71 Schiavi RC, Schreiner-Engel P, Mandeli J, Schanzer H, Cohen E: Healthy aging and male sexual function. Am J Psychiatry 1990;147:766–771.
72 Kaplan HS: Anxiety and sexual dysfunction. J Clin Psychiatry 1988;49:21–25.
73 Fossey MD, Hamner MB: Clonazepam-related sexual dysfunction in male veterans with PTSD. Anxiety 1994–1995;1:233–236.
74 Kotler M, Cohen H, Aizenberg D, Matar M, Loewenthal U, Kaplan Z, Miodownik H, Zemishlany Z: Sexual dysfunction in male posttraumatic stress disorder patients. Psychother Psychosom 2000; 69:309–315.
75 Horowitz M, Wilner N, Alvarez W: Impact of Event Scale: a measure of subjective stress. Psychosom Med 1979;41:209–218.
76 Derogatis L, Cleary P: A confirmation of dimensional structure of the SCL-90: A study in construct validity. J Clin Psychiatry 1977;33:981–989.
77 Reznik I, Zemishlany Z, Kotler M, Spivak B, Weizman A, Mester R: Sildenafil citrate for the sexual dysfunction in antidepressant-treated male patients with posttraumatic stress disorder. A preliminary pilot open-label study. Psychother Psychosom 2002;71:173–176.
78 Raboch J: Sexual development and life of psychiatric female patients. Arch Sex Bahav 1986;15:341–353.
79 Raboch J, Faltus F: Sexuality of women with anorexia nervosa. Acta Psychiatr Scand 1991;84: 9–11.
80 Simpson WS, Ramberg JA: Sexual dysfunction in married female patients with anorexia and bulimia nervosa. J Sex Marital Ther 1992;18:44–45.

81 Tuiten A, Panhuysen G, Everaerd W, Koppeschaar H, Drabbe P, Zelissen P: The paradoxical nature of sexuality in anorexia nervosa. J Sex Marital Ther 1993;19:259–275.

82 Morgan CD: Sexual functioning and attitudes of eating-disordered women: A follow-up study. J Sex Marital Ther 1995;21:67–77.

83 Zanarini MC, Parachini EA, Frankenburg FR, Holman JB, Hennen J, Bradford Reich D, Silk KR: Sexual relationship difficulties among borderline patients and axis II comparison subjects. J Nerv Ment Dis 2003;191:479–482.

Prof. Zvi Zemishlany
Geha Mental Health Center
1 Helsinki Street, PO Box 102
IL–49100 Petah-Tikva (Israel)
Tel. +972 3 925 8205, Fax +972 3 924 1941, E-Mail zzemishlany@clalit.org.il

Balon R (ed): Sexual Dysfunction. The Brain-Body Connection.
Adv Psychosom Med. Basel, Karger, 2008, vol 29, pp 107–130

Psychotropics and Sexual Dysfunction: The Evidence and Treatments

Lawrence A. Labbate

Department of Psychiatry, University of Arkansas for Medical Sciences, Little Rock, Ark., USA

Abstract

Sexual dysfunction is common in the general population and even more common in the mentally or medically ill. Because mentally ill patients often receive psychotropics, many of which affect sexual functioning, a patient's pre-existing sexual difficulties are often compounded, and these adverse effects may contribute to psychological difficulties or medication discontinuation. The effects of antidepressants, antipsychotics, mood stabilizers and anxiolytics on sexual functioning are critically reviewed. When possible, the types of sexual dysfunction (e.g. desire, arousal, or orgasm) induced by the drug is described. Treatments for drug-induced sexual function are described, but few controlled studies show benefit. Only sildenafil stands as a convincing treatment for drug-induced sexual dysfunction. The paper focuses on the placebo-controlled clinical trials that specifically evaluated sexual functioning in patients treated with psychotropics. Controlled studies are few for all the agents, though best for the antidepressants and antipsychotics. The exact magnitude and phase of sexual functioning affected remains to be elucidated for most psychotropic drugs. Although all phases of sexual functioning may be impaired by psychotropics, selective serotonin reuptake inhibitor antidepressants appear to primarily affect orgasm, while antipsychotics primarily affect desire. There is insufficient evidence to make conclusions about the anxiolytics or mood stabilizers.

Sexual dysfunction is common in the general population and even more common in the mentally or medically ill. Because mentally ill patients are often prescribed psychotropics, many of which are well known to affect sexual functioning, a patient's pre-existing sexual difficulties are often compounded, and these adverse effects may contribute to psychological difficulties or medication discontinuation. Because psychotropics may ameliorate seriously debilitating illnesses, such as depressive disorders or schizophrenia, stopping medication may have profound negative effects, such as job loss or marital disruption. It is therefore critical to understand the effects of psychotropics on sexual function in the mentally ill and to make use of this information in prescribing patients psychotropics.

Although some aspects of psychotropic-associated sexual dysfunction are understood, unfortunately many are not. Clinical trials evaluating sexual function often exclude patients with systemic medical problems or multiple medications that could affect sexual functioning. Parsing the effect of the mental illness and the psychotropics on sexual function is also not well established and may be impossible. Sexual functioning or sexual well-being is complex, with multiple contributing psychological, interpersonal, and medical factors. For example, serotonin reuptake antidepressants are frequently prescribed for depressed patients with coronary artery disease following myocardial infarction or cardiac surgery. With so many possible contributors to sexual dysfunction (e.g. peripheral vascular disease, cardiac medications, depression, marital problems, antidepressant use), isolating the effect of one variable, such as a single psychotropic, is unrealistic. Hence, the state of the art is derived from patients with uncomplicated disorders, usually taking just one medication.

Furthermore, because sexual function or dysfunction is difficult to measure, the meaning of the findings is sometimes difficult to interpret. A person's description of sexual functioning is likely affected by perception of social norms and may have a common variation influenced by relationships and cultural factors. Rating scales may be inefficient in detecting subtle differences that are highly subjective. Although there are numerous rating scales, usually with expanded items related to sexual interest, genital arousal, orgasm, and overall satisfaction, none is uniformly employed, thereby making comparisons between drugs difficult. Even the so-called validated rating instruments, when used in clinical trials of psychotropics, produce findings with small changes of marginal importance, such as mild delay in orgasm, a sometimes welcome effect for men. When changes in sexual functioning are in the mild range, the findings are of questionable clinical validity because it is difficult to know if these changes are related to the normal fluctuation of sexual function, the illness being treated, or the effects of drugs. Thus, only categorical findings (e.g. inability to attain orgasm) or truly measured effects (e.g. minutes to reach orgasm) may have true face validity.

Clinical trials specifically addressing sexual functioning rarely have a placebo control group. Hence, little is known about the sexual effects of the antidepressants compared with placebo. Placebo-controlled studies may not force questions about sexual functioning, but often rely on spontaneous reports, which are well known to be less forthcoming than direct inquiry. Most large studies are drug company-sponsored, and those specifically addressing sexual functioning are often sponsored by the company whose drug is suspected to have fewer sexual side effects. These studies may report small differences that are statistically significant, but of uncertain clinical difference, and these studies ordinarily do not include a placebo group.

Most importantly, studies generally do not address premorbid sexual functioning. Because it is well known that mental illnesses affect sexual functioning and disrupt interpersonal relationships, it is very difficult to ascribe sexual difficulties to illness or the drug. These two factors, of course, are not the only contributors to sexual functioning, for systemic illness and substance abuse also accompany patients with mental illness and further complicate the conundrum. An ideal study to address the effects of drugs on sexual functioning would measure sexual functioning in physically healthy patients before the illness started and then prospectively follow the changes in sexual functioning following the start of the drug. In addition, a control sample would be needed to determine how much variability could be attributed to the natural course of being in drug treatment for a mental illness.

Cross-sectional comparison studies of psychotropics avoid the issue of the effects of disease and drug. In these studies, it is impossible to determine if it is the drug or the disease that is responsible for a person's sexual dysfunction. Without randomization or a comparison sample taking placebo, it is impossible to know the contributions of a drug to a person's reported sexual problems. In the cross-sectional design, isolating the effects of a drug on sexual functioning is nearly impossible because preexisting conditions could certainly be culpable for the current difficulties, even though attempts are made to retrospectively isolate the drug effect from long-standing psychological factors, the effects of psychiatric illness, occult substance abuse, or undiagnosed medical conditions.

With these limitations in mind, this chapter will review the clinical effects of psychotropics on sexual functioning and what, if anything, can be done to treat adverse effects associated with psychotropic medications. Emphasis will be placed on those randomized, placebo-controlled clinical trials in which sexual functioning was specifically evaluated with a rating instrument. Because these are relatively few, other comparison and naturalistic clinical trials will also be addressed. Most psychotropic studies evaluating sexual dysfunction concern antidepressants, though there is a reasonable body of evidence regarding antipsychotics, and a much smaller literature about mood stabilizers, and anxiolytics.

The effects of antidepressants, antipsychotics, mood stabilizers and anxiolytics on sexual functioning will be reviewed. When possible, the types of sexual dysfunction (e.g. desire, arousal, or orgasm) induced by the drug will be described. Additionally, treatments to alleviate psychotropic-associated sexual dysfunction will be detailed, but there is, unfortunately, precious little controlled data about how to effectively treat drug-induced sexual problems. Until effective psychotropic medications are discovered that do not affect sexual functioning, coping with these vexing problems remains a challenge.

Antidepressants

Many patients suffering from mood disorders have sexual difficulties. Studies suggest that at least half of patients will have some aspect of sexual functioning affected. Loss of interest and social withdrawal may have profound influences on the ability to maintain intimate relationships. Although loss of interest in sex is probably the most common aspect of sexual dysfunction [1], depressive disorders may also affect arousal, and orgasm, the same three parameters that many antidepressants affect. Mood disorders may lead to loss of interest in sex, emotional withdrawal from a love interest, and subsequent performance anxiety about having sex. Hence, unless clinicians take detailed sexual histories at the start of antidepressant treatment, and ideally before mental disorders begin, separating the sexual difficulties of the mood disorder from those induced by the antidepressant is difficult, if not impossible. In addition to loss of desire, arousal or orgasm dysfunction associated with a depressive disorder, patients may also have pre-existing sexual problems (e.g. premature ejaculation or anorgasmia) and medical problems (e.g. diabetes, peripheral vascular disease, or ischemic heart disease) that may compromise sexual functioning. Even though patients may have multiple factors contributing to sexual dysfunction, patients appear reluctant to volunteer sexual information to clinicians, and physicians may be reluctant to ask about sexual matters. Not surprisingly, studies find that patients are far more likely to report sexual difficulties when they are directly queried rather than when the clinicians give them the chance for an unprompted response [2, 3].

Until recent years, studies of antidepressants did not specifically address sexual side effects and relied completely on self-report. This led to low reported rates of sexual dysfunction. For example, the initial PDR rate for fluoxetine-associated sexual effects was 1.9%, though many studies later found rates to be between 30–40% of patients.

Serotonin Reuptake Inhibitors

The selective serotonin reuptake inhibitors (SSRIs) are a group of antidepressants that increase the availability of serotonin in the synapse via inhibition of the serotonin transporter. For this review, SSRIs will refer to the usual medication grouping (fluoxetine, citalopram, escitalopram, paroxetine, sertraline, and fluvoxamine) as well as the two drugs that inhibit serotonin and norepinephrine reuptake (venlafaxine and duloxetine).

Although serotonin's effects on sexual behavior are complex and not fully elucidated in animal models, in general, increased synaptic serotonin has an inhibitory effect on sexual functioning. The individual SSRI agents vary slightly in their pharmacologic profiles, with a range of potency at the serotonin transporter, and some have effects on other receptor sites that may influence sexual functioning. For example, fluoxetine mildly inhibits norepinephrine reuptake, while sertraline modestly blocks reuptake of dopamine. Paroxetine, perhaps the most problematic of the SSRIs for sexual function, slightly blocks postsynaptic dopamine type 2 receptors and also inhibits nitric oxide oxidase activity, thereby affecting sexual function by multiple mechanisms.

Even though the SSRIs have a clear reputation for affecting sexual functioning, there are relatively few placebo-controlled prospective studies carefully evaluating sexual effects of the SSRIs. Because sexual problems are common in the general population as well as in depressed individuals [4], it remains somewhat difficult to fully ascribe the sexual effects associated with depression treatment solely to antidepressants. Moreover, different rating scales are used in the studies, and there are no prospective randomized placebo-controlled studies comparing all of the SSRIs.

Nonetheless, the limited number of prospective studies investigating individual SSRI drugs in depressed patients suggests that the SSRI antidepressants are generally similar in their propensity to affect sexual function. There is no evidence that one SSRI is superior to another. Although all aspects of sexual functioning are affected, including libido, arousal and orgasm, there is some suggestion that delayed orgasm is the most commonly affected sexual parameter. In many studies, however, the magnitude of change is relatively small and it is difficult to determine the clinical relevance of the sexual change and to dissect the drug effect from the depression effect on sexual function.

In the last 5 years, a few studies have been specifically performed to evaluate sexual function with antidepressants. There have been a number of pharmaceutical company studies sponsored by manufacturers of mirtazapine or bupropion, attempting to show their relative benefit for sexual side effects compared with SSRI antidepressants. These studies have shown some advantages, but they are not overwhelming. Studies that specifically evaluated sexual function are reviewed below.

In a short-term study comparing venlafaxine (mean dose 150 mg) with bupropion (mean dose 300 mg) for depression (n = 328), sexual function was rated over the course of the study with a validated rating scale [5]. In the depressed patients with so called normal sexual functioning at the start of antidepressant treatment (n = 251), the authors found that patients treated with venlafaxine fared less well than those treated with bupropion in all aspects of sexual functioning. This difference between treatments was statistically significant, but the change in magnitude was quite small (three points, with a baseline score over 42 for women and 48 for men), making it difficult to determine if the change was clinically significant. Moreover, the change on individual items (pleasure, desire, arousal and orgasm) was less than a point. Although the authors, funded by the manufacturers of bupropion, concluded that bupropion 'had a significantly more favorable sexual side effect profile' than venlafaxine, the data suggest a small advantage. The study's findings were limited by the lack of a placebo comparison group.

In a study (n = 345) comparing sertraline with mirtazapine for rate of onset of antidepressant effect, sexual effects of mirtazapine and sertraline were also studied prospectively [6]. This was a usual clinical trial sample that excluded patients with systemic medical conditions, many of which also affect sexual functioning. As with the bupropion and venlafaxine study listed above, the difference between the two groups with regard to sexual functioning was quite small. The study found no overall differences between groups on depression symptoms, and very minor, though statistically significant changes on a sexual rating scale. Interestingly, there is some evidence of *improvement* in sexual functioning over the course of the study in both groups, with somewhat higher rates attaining normal sexual function in the mirtazapine group than the sertraline group. Without a placebo comparison group, a limited number of conclusions can be drawn, though it appears that in this sample of patients the sexual side effects were relatively modest. The authors, funded by the manufacturer of mirtazapine, however, concluded that 'mirtazapine had a greater effect than sertraline on sexual functioning'.

In a placebo-controlled study (n = 456) evaluating bupropion and fluoxetine for depression [7], patients were specifically questioned whether several parameters of sexual functioning (orgasm, desire, or arousal) were present or absent, and if the sexual parameter was rated as 'better', 'no change' or 'worse' than baseline. Hence, this study primarily measured if a problem was present or absent and did not measure severity on a graded rating scale. Over the course of the study, the percent of patients with sexual desire problems did not change in the fluoxetine or placebo groups, though the problematic percent dropped in the bupropion group (25–10%). Sexual arousal, however, worsened in approximately 10% in the fluoxetine and placebo groups and was no different from bupropion. Only in orgasm dysfunction was there a clear difference between fluoxetine, placebo, and bupropion. For orgasm dysfunction, approximately 30% of the fluoxetine patients reported orgasm difficulty; while only 10% of placebo- and bupropion-treated patients experienced this problem. This study, more than others, demonstrated that orgasm is the principal sexual function affected by fluoxetine.

A careful study evaluating bupropion and sertraline (again, without a placebo group) [8] funded by the manufactures of bupropion, took into account sexual functioning problems at the start of antidepressant treatment. The authors found that sertraline was associated with more sexual problems than bupropion. At the start of the study, however, 43% of patients in both groups were not satisfied with their sexual functioning. Following treatment, the percent of sertraline-treated patients that were unsatisfied did not change, but the bupropion treated patients fared better, with only 21% reporting that they were unsatisfied. Both groups improved similarly with respect to depression. Comparing groups according to rates of dissatisfaction is somewhat difficult to appreciate, but overall, it is reasonable to conclude that bupropion helped reverse sexual dysfunction as depression remitted, but sertraline did not improve sexual functioning as patients' mood increased. Additionally, orgasm dysfunction (defined as delay and/or failure) was far more common with sertraline than bupropion (52 vs. 8%), but the magnitude of this dysfunction was not delineated. That is, it was not reported how many of the patients had orgasm failure and how many were only delayed. In some cases, particularly for men, delay in orgasm would not be of serious consequence. Thus, although the difference between the two drugs appears impressive, it is not certain that the difference was of meaningful clinical significance.

In a study comparing fluoxetine (n = 150) with reboxetine (n = 150) and placebo (n = 150) in depressed patients [9], overall sexual satisfaction was relatively low at the start of treatment (mean score approximately 35 on a visual analogue scale from 0 to 100), and following treatment there was a relatively small increase (7 points) in sexual satisfaction in the placebo group compared to a small decrease (4 points) in the fluoxetine group. Although this difference was statistically significant, the clinical relevance is marginal, and, overall, patients were still rating their overall sexual satisfaction score at a low level. Fluoxetine was similar to placebo on several dichotomous items regarding sexual functioning, though fluoxetine-treated patients were more likely than placebo-treated patients to endorse that 'more stimulation was needed to attain an erection than usual' (42 vs. 21%).

Finally, in a pooled analysis of 1,477 patients enrolled in studies sponsored by the manufacturer of duloxetine that compared duloxetine (40–120 mg/day) with paroxetine (20 mg/day) and placebo [10], investigators found that paroxetine was associated with sexual dysfunction more frequently than duloxetine or placebo. Of note, 59% of the patients reported significant sexual dysfunction at the start of drug treatment as measured by a brief questionnaire. Among 475 patients who completed baseline and endpoint rating scales and 'did not report significant sexual difficulties with sex drive, arousal, or orgasm at baseline', there were considerable treatment-emergent sexual adverse effects following treatment. The definition of sexual dysfunction was quite wide, ranging from patients with 'somewhat difficult troubles' to 'inability to get aroused or have orgasm'. The incidence of newly acquired sexual dysfunction was as follows: paroxetine 61%, duloxetine 46%, and placebo 29%. This suggests that although duloxetine may be somewhat less problematic than paroxetine, there remains considerable risk for sexual dysfunction, albeit for a range of impairment. For the patients who developed more severe sexual dysfunction (rated as 'very difficult' to 'never have orgasm or arousal') there were differences only in the orgasm dimension. The presence of serious orgasm difficulties following treatment were as follows: paroxetine 20%, duloxetine 16%, placebo 9%. Both drugs led to serious orgasm difficulties more than placebo and there were no differences between the two antidepressants for this more serious adverse effect. In all, it appears that duloxetine frequently caused minor sexual problems, at slightly higher rates than paroxetine, but duloxetine was just as likely to cause significant orgasm difficulties as low-dose paroxetine.

Mirtazapine

Mirtazapine is commonly reported to induce less sexual dysfunction than serotonin reuptake antidepressants, though it has not been specifically studied in placebo-controlled trials for this property. Naturalistic, cross-sectional studies find that mirtazapine is either associated with lower or similar rates of sexual side effects compared with serotonin reuptake inhibitors. In these nonrandomized studies, little is known about pretreatment sexual functioning or how drugs were chosen. It could be that patients were selected for mirtazapine because of its theoretical lower incidence of sexual dysfunction, but without randomization or a control group it is difficult to know in naturalistic studies the true extent of drug-induced side effects. If patients were selected because they were concerned about sexual functioning, then this bias might influence the results. One large cross-sectional study found that 24% of patients treated with mirtazapine reported sexual side effects compared with 60–70% of patients treated with serotonin reuptake inhibitors [11].

Although prospective studies evaluating sexual function are lacking, a few small studies produce information from which it can be deduced that sexual dysfunction is limited with mirtazapine. In a study (n = 24) of men with premature ejaculation, mirtazapine proved of no benefit in delaying ejaculations, so it can be reasonably deduced that mirtazapine may not cause orgasm delay in depressed men [12].

In a naturalistic trial (n = 19), patients with SSRI-associated sexual dysfunction, whose depression was remitted, were switched to mirtazapine [13]. Patients continued to do well with regard to their mood following the medication switch, and, over the study period, 58% of patients had reversal of their sexual dysfunction. This change was impressive, though 17% of patients gained 10–20 pounds, thereby making this option a questionable trade-off. The true effects of mirtazapine on sexual functioning in depressed individuals remain to be tested.

Nefazodone

Although nefazodone has the reputation of causing low rates of sexual problems, principally because of its lack of enhancing serotonin transmission and blocking 5-HT2 receptors, it has not been specifically studied for its sexual effects in prospective placebo controlled trials. In a comparison study with sertraline (n = 72), nefazodone-treated patients (n = 71) fared better than sertraline-treated patients with respect to orgasm, but not arousal [14]. Far more sertraline patients complained of difficulty attaining orgasm with sertraline (67%) than with nefazodone (19%). Patients received clinically relevant doses of both drugs; mean daily dose of sertraline was approximately 150 mg, and the mean dose of nefazodone was approximately 450 mg. Hence, although the data are limited, it appears that nefazodone has a low rate of causing sexual problems. The original manufacturer of nefazodone unfortunately stopped making the drug because of its rare association with severe hepatic toxicity. Although available from a generic pharmaceutical company, the drug is rarely prescribed now.

Treatment of SSRI-Associated Sexual Dysfunction

There are several ways to approach treatment of sexual dysfunction associated with SSRI antidepressants. As mentioned before, it is critical to determine sexual functioning before the start of treatment and to consider the contribution of medical, psychological and interpersonal factors that may be contributing to sexual difficulties. These factors will help guide treatment. With this in mind, for the patient in whom sexual functioning is essential, the choice of a drug with limited proclivity to cause sexual problems makes good sense. Bupropion, mirtazapine or nefazodone would make reasonable choices to minimize antidepressant-induced side effects.

Briefly stopping offending antidepressants has been proposed as a technique for reversing sexual problems associated with antidepressants, though this method has not been extensively studied, and the benefits appear only for approximately half of patients with shorter-acting SSRIs (sertraline, paroxetine and fluvoxamine), but not for patients with longer-acting drugs such as fluoxetine. The other problem with briefly stopping the antidepressants is that patients may experience a withdrawal syndrome or the return of the anxiety or depression symptoms that were the initial targets for medication treatment. In all, this drug-holiday method appears of limited value, with the risks likely greater than the benefits. Although this method may be useful for a selected group of patients, perhaps those with less severe conditions, the characteristics of the patients for whom this would be useful have not been elucidated.

Switching from a serotonin reuptake inhibitor to an agent somewhat less likely to cause sexual dysfunction, such as bupropion or nefazodone, is another reasonable option for combating SSRI-associated sexual dysfunction. This method, though logical, has not been studied in randomized controlled trials.

There have been several small open-label studies showing improvement in sexual functioning in patients switched to bupropion. In small samples, bupropion appears to be an effective option for remitted, depressed patients who are switched from fluoxetine to bupropion or from several SSRIs to mirtazapine. Switching medications to evaluate the benefits on sexual functioning has not been studied in controlled fashion in patients who experience partially treated depression. Some patients who are intolerant of SSRIs may respond to mirtazapine, bupropion or nefazodone, and they may benefit from the reduced sexual side effect burden compared with the SSRIs. The potential pitfall of this approach is that some patients may lose the benefit of the SSRI when they are switched to a non-SSRI antidepressant. Moreover, patients switched to mirtazapine may develop significant weight gain that could be an unsatisfactory side effect exchange. Although some patients may be less prone toward sexual side effects from one SSRI compared with another, this method has not been systematically studied.

A number of agents have been reported to be useful to reverse the deleterious sexual effects of antidepressants. Despite the many positive open-label case reports of successful treatments with the addition of medications (including amantadine, dextroamphetamine, cyproheptadine, pramipexole), only a few treatments have proven benefit, and, of those, some show only modest benefit in placebo-controlled trials. Bupropion has been used for a number of years as an adjunct for treating partially responsive depression or for reversing sexual dysfunction. Despite early reports of its benefit for sexual dysfunction in open-label trials [15], it appears that bupropion's benefit may only occur at relatively high doses (300 mg per day) [16] because the addition of lower doses (150 mg per day) prove no more effective than placebo, and the benefits at the higher doses may only benefit libido.

The addition of higher-dose bupropion to SSRIs, unfortunately, may lead to new untoward side effects, especially anxiety or irritability, thus sometimes making the combination intolerable and therefore ineffective for its intended purpose of relieving sexual problems.

Similarly, early optimistic reports of the benefits of the addition of buspirone to antidepressants for resolving sexual dysfunction were quieted when relatively low doses (30 mg per day) added to SSRIs proved no better than placebo in ameliorating SSRI-associated sexual dysfunction. On the other hand, the addition of higher doses of buspirone (50–60 mg) to patients who were taking citalopram or paroxetine for depression proved effective for sexual dysfunction [17]. In this study, 40% of patients taking the SSRI antidepressant developed some sort of sexual dysfunction (arousal, interest or orgasm), and these patients (n = 47) were randomized to the addition of buspirone or placebo. By the study end, patients taking buspirone fared convincingly better than the placebo-treated patients, with nearly twice as many patients taking buspirone reporting remittance in sexual problems compared with placebo-treated patients (58 vs. 30%). The benefit was greater in women than in men, and, interestingly, the benefit came within the 1st week, persisted, and did not change over the 4-week study. It is not known if longer treatment leads to continued benefit. The addition of buspirone was well tolerated, though unfortunately did not improve depressive symptoms compared with placebo. This beneficial effect on sexual functioning, if replicated in a larger sample, suggests that the addition of buspirone is a relatively benign treatment option in which results will be quickly known.

The only conclusively effective treatment for sexual problems associated with SSRIs is for the addition of sildenafil for antidepressant-induced erectile dysfunction. Add-on studies, unfortunately, have only been conducted in men whose depression was in remission, though there are some interesting findings that in men with mild depression, sildenafil alone, without antidepressant treatment, may improve erectile dysfunction and lead to modest mood improvement [18].

Two placebo-controlled add-on studies show clear evidence that sildenafil improves SSRI antidepressant-induced erectile problems, and that sildenafil may, to a lesser degree, improve other aspects of sexual dysfunction as well [19, 20]. In these flexibly dosed studies, the addition of sildenafil (25–100 mg) to SSRI antidepressants showed clear improvement in the ability to attain a satisfactory erection and have sexual intercourse. Interestingly, although erectile dysfunction was the requirement to enter the study, men also experienced sexual dysfunction in other domains (interest, orgasm, overall satisfaction) and sildenafil helped improve each area, though the benefit was obvious for erectile dysfunction and more modest in the other areas. Of note, sildenafil was well tolerated and there was no loss of antidepressant benefit with the addition of sildenafil to the SSRI antidepressants. Although controlled studies show benefit up to 100 mg, open-label anecdotal experience suggest some men may require doses up to 200 mg to reverse SSRI-associated erectile dysfunction.

Antidepressant Summary

The SSRI antidepressants, though commonly known to cause sexual dysfunction, have had only limited prospective study evaluating sexual function, and few of these studies have had placebo comparisons. In the relatively healthy patients enrolled in the SSRI trials, orgasm appears to be the most commonly affected sexual function, perhaps being reduced in 30–40% of patients, though the magnitude of the side effect may not always be serious. Likely because sexual problems are very common in the general population, point prevalence studies in patients taking antidepressants show higher rates of sexual dysfunction than prospective studies. Other non-SSRI antidepressants such as bupropion or nefazodone may cause somewhat lower rates of sexual dysfunction than the SSRIs, but the advantage may be primarily with the effects on orgasm. The only established effective antidote for SSRI-associated sexual dysfunction is sildenafil for the treatment of SSRI-induced erectile dysfunction.

Antipsychotics

Sexual dysfunction in patients with schizophrenia has been ignored until recent years. Although clinicians or investigators may have assumed that sexual activity was unimportant or not practiced in this population, this proved not to be the case. Moreover, patients with schizophrenia rarely report sexual dysfunction spontaneously, and it was therefore initially, if blindly, reported that sexual dysfunction was uncommon in antipsychotic clinical trials. More careful attention to this sexual adverse effect revealed that direct questioning about sexual side effects led to the realization that sexual side effects were common problems of the antipsychotics. Psychiatrists, however, continue to underestimate the presence of sexual dysfunction in their patients with schizophrenia [21]. As with depressed patients taking antidepressants, patients with schizophrenia underreport sexual side effects associated with antipsychotics. Patients are more likely to report sexual side effects when they are directly questioned.

Sexual side effects, in fact, appear to be very disconcerting to patients with psychotic disorders and may be an important reason for medication discontent or medication noncompliance. Recognizing the degree of sexual side effects associated with the antipsychotics is particularly important because antipsychotic use has extended well beyond patients with schizophrenia.

Sexual problems in patients with psychotic disorders is complex, with contributions from the primary illness (lack of motivation, poor interpersonal relationships), weight gain, smoking, drug or alcohol abuse, and medication side effects. The antipsychotic drugs may contribute to sexual side dysfunction by antagonizing cholinergic receptors, adrenergic receptors or dopamine receptors. Antipsychotic drugs may lead to sedation, loss of interest, or loss of erections. Although the exact mechanism of antipsychotic-induced sexual dysfunction is not fully elucidated, the presumed primary cause of sexual dysfunction is related to the drugs blocking dopamine receptors in the anterior pituitary and thereby causing hyperprolactinemia. Elevated prolactin in the plasma may then lead to galactorrhea, breast enlargement, decreased libido, anorgasmia and erectile dysfunction. Other central nervous system or peripheral effects may be responsible, but these are not elucidated.

The first-generation antipsychotics, particularly the high-potency drugs such as fluphenazine or haloperidol, seemingly lead to more adverse sexual side effects than the second-generation antipsychotics, though there is limited study comparing the various drugs. The second-generation antipsychotics may be less prone to cause sexual side effects because they block serotonin 5-HT2 receptors, though this is not established. The one clear exception to the second-generation antipsychotics being less problematic for sexual side effects is risperidone, presumably because it elevates prolactin similar to the first-generation antipsychotics. Among the older antipsychotics, thioridazine is of note because of its capacity to cause retrograde ejaculation. Haloperidol or fluphenazine is historically associated with erectile failure.

As with the antidepressants, there are numerous difficulties in appraising the effect of the drugs on sexual functioning. Parsing the effect of the antipsychotic medication, psychotic illness, depressive symptoms, drug or alcohol use, and contributing medical conditions (e.g. smoking or diabetes) is very difficult. There are numerous rating scales and it is unknown how valid they are in patients with schizophrenia. Most studies, moreover, do not report sexual functioning before medication treatment, and evaluating sexual function before the onset of the psychotic illness is likely impossible. Many investigations into the effects of sexual function are not randomized, and sample sizes are generally quite small in the few controlled studies. There are, unfortunately, no placebo-controlled prospective studies evaluating sexual dysfunction with antipsychotics. Hence, the quality of the information remains limited, but there is clear indication that the antipsychotics do cause sexual problems that may need attention. Interestingly, although the antipsychotics are used across many diagnoses, the limited data pertain primarily to patients with schizophrenia. There is very little information regarding the adverse sexual side effects of the antipsychotics in patients with bipolar disorder or other conditions.

Though there are no placebo-controlled randomized clinical trials specifically evaluating drug-induced sexual effects, there are several comparison and naturalistic studies. One small study (n = 27, 85% male) [22] evaluated patients with treatment-refractory schizophrenia following a 4–6 week lead-in with first generation antipsychotics. The questionnaire was administered following the lead-in medication, and then patients were randomized to a 12-week trial of risperidone (4 mg/day), quetiapine (400 mg/day) or fluphenazine (12.5 mg/day). The rating scale measured 'any trouble maintaining an erection, painful prolonged erections, troubled ejaculating when wanted, loss of interest once aroused, and/or not able to have an orgasm if wanted'. The authors primarily reported the presence of sexual dysfunction rather than the degree of sexual dysfunction using a rating scale with very low threshold for establishing sexual dysfunction. The study was not designed with sexual function as the primary outcome, rather it was primarily designed to evaluate efficacy of second-generation antipsychotics in treatment-resistant patients. Because it was designed for reasons other than evaluating sexual side effects, the lead-in treatment with various antipsychotics poses a clear confound. Additionally, patients could receive lorazepam, benztropine or propranolol, all of which could contribute to sexual side effects. Lastly, there was no placebo control to serve as a comparison.

These limitations understood, the study found that patients treated with fluphenazine were more likely than risperidone- or quetiapine-treated patients to report sexual dysfunction. As measured with this very sensitive rating scale, all groups experienced high rates of sexual dysfunction: fluphenazine 78%, quetiapine 50% and risperidone 42%. Examining items that contribute to the total rating scale score reveals that mean scores at baseline were in the dysfunctional range, perhaps related to the lead-in treatment, and endpoint changed very little in any of the groups. Only in the quetiapine-treated patients was there some improvement over the course of the trial, and this was only of clinical significance in the area of arousal/erection. Asked if there was any improvement over the course of the trial, patients treated with fluphenazine uncommonly reported this benefit, whereas approximately half of the risperidone- and quetiapine-treated patients reported improvement. The degree of this sexual improvement was not reported, though the change in the sexual function subsections of the questionnaire suggest that this change was small, and the change was likely due to the switch from a first generation antipsychotic to the second generation drug. Thus, the benefits attained from quetiapine treatment may have been due primarily from stopping the pretreatment first-generation antipsychotic. Indeed, for quetiapine there was a considerable drop in prolactin concentration over the course of the study (range –17 to –59 mg/dl). The small sample size and that the patients were treatment nonresponders limits the generalization of the data. The authors concluded that quetiapine had the greatest benefit among the drugs regarding sexual functioning. This may be true, but the benefit was modest.

Another study evaluated 46 patients (80% male, mean age 27) with a psychotic disorder who were openly switched from a previous antipsychotic to risperidone or olanzapine when they entered the study [23]. Patients were switched off their previous medication because of clinical need, usually worsened psychosis, and the previous medication could not be risperidone or olanzapine. Patients were not told that the primary interest of the study was to evaluate sexual functioning. Patients were followed for 6 weeks and sexual dysfunction was assessed by a sexual function questionnaire and a side effect rating scale after 6 weeks. Patients were queried regarding libido, erection, ejaculation and orgasm. Unfortunately, and this is a significant limitation of the study, baseline sexual functioning was not recorded, thereby limiting the interpretation of the data because it is not known if sexual dysfunction existed prior to starting the antipsychotic.

Patients took only risperidone (n = 21) or olanzapine (n = 25), and mean doses at the time of evaluation for sexual functioning were olanzapine 9.4 mg/day and risperidone 3.4 mg/day. In both groups, the degree of psychosis improvement was similar. Sexual function, however, was more impaired in the risperidone- than the olanzapine-treated patients. Using categorical values (any to severe) to determine the presence of sexual dysfunction, 52% of risperidone-treated patients and 12% of olanzapine-treated patients reported sexual dysfunction. Even though they rated severity of symptoms on a three-point scale (absent, some problems, many problems), the authors did not specify the severity of the sexual dysfunction, though they noted that patients using risperidone 'experienced more serious problems'. All aspects of sexual functioning were similarly impaired. Erections were impaired in 32% of men taking risperidone, but not in any of the men taking olanzapine. Of note, only 9% of patients spontaneously reported sexual difficulties.

This small study, limited as it is by the lack of a placebo and baseline measurements, suggests that olanzapine may be less problematic than risperidone for causing sexual side effects, but further controlled study with baseline measurements are needed to confirm this possibility.

A small short-term study (n = 22, all men) found that blindly switching from risperidone to quetiapine (mean dose 300 mg) or continuing with risperidone (mean dose 4.3 mg) provided no benefit in sexual functioning as measured on a 5-item questionnaire for patients who experienced sexual dysfunction while taking risperidone [24].

The authors found that there was a modest correlation between prolactin levels and rating scale scores in the risperidone, but not the quetiapine groups, but it is unclear if this correlation is of any clinical meaning because there was no difference between groups in overall sexual function. The sample size was not powered to find a difference. Larger samples may reveal different results.

Point Prevalence Studies

A point prevalence investigation of sexual side effects in patients (n = 636) with schizophrenia was conducted in Spain [25]. This study evaluated if there were differences among antipsychotics with respect to sexual functioning. Because the study was nonrandom and included other medications, the findings are limited. The authors, nonetheless, found that nearly 40% of patients experienced some sort of sexual dysfunction. Without baseline measures, it is unknown how much of this effect was drug related or if sexual functioning before the start of medication influenced physicians in choosing an antipsychotic. They found that rates of sexual dysfunction were lower in quetiapine (18%) compared with haloperidol (38%), olanzapine (38%) or risperidone (42%). Because there was no randomization, the differences among the antipsychotics may be due to factors other than medication.

A recent naturalistic examination of sexual dysfunction in a Turkish study evaluated point prevalence of sexual dysfunction in 827 stabilized outpatients with schizophrenia. The authors found that just over 50% of patients experienced sexual dysfunction [26].

Sexual problems were present to a similar degree in desire, orgasm and arousal. Not surprisingly, smoking compounded the effects of antipsychotics on sexual functioning. Patients taking multiple medications experience more severe sexual side effects than patients taking a single second-generation antipsychotic.

Another recent, though smaller, point prevalence American study (n = 238) [27] also found high rates of considerable sexual dysfunction in patients with schizophrenia, and while there were slightly lower mean scores on a sexual function rating scale for quetiapine-treated patients compared with those taking olanzapine or risperidone, the difference was small and of doubtful clinical importance. Without baseline, predrug treatment sexual function measurements, all that can be said is that sexual dysfunction is common in patients with schizophrenia treated with antipsychotics.

A large international naturalistic study of patients diagnosed with schizophrenia receiving 3 months of monotherapy antipsychotics (n = 3,838), funded by the manufacturer of olanzapine, compared sexual function in patients treated with one of four antipsychotics [28]. In this 3-year prospective study, patients with schizophrenia were treated with an antipsychotic of the clinician's choice, but for unstated reasons more than half of the patients (n = 2,638) received olanzapine as their first drug. For the other groups, the number of patients was considerably smaller: risperidone, n = 860; quetiapine, n = 142; haloperidol, n = 188. Patients were included in the analysis if they stayed on a single antipsychotic medication for at least 3 months. Mean doses for the agents were fairly typical for outpatients: olanzapine 11 mg, risperidone 4 mg, quetiapine 340 mg, haloperidol 11 mg.

Sexual function was measured according to patient reports and psychiatrist perception at visits conducted at 3, 6, and 12 months following start of treatment. Psychiatrists rated items of sexual function according to a side effect-rating scale as either present, absent or not applicable. These ratings were to evaluate the presence or absence of loss of libido, amenorrhea, gynecomastia, impotence, or galactorrhea. Additionally, patients completed a separate written evaluation in which they reported if their sexual function was 'no problem', 'some problem' or 'unable to perform sexually'. Because many patients had sexual dysfunction at baseline, only patients without symptoms at baseline were included in the analysis to determine treatment-emergent symptoms.

For the total sample, sexual problems were very common with all the antipsychotics. During the 12-month study period, the proportion of patients reporting any sexual dysfunction was as follows: haloperidol (71%); risperidone (68%); quetiapine (60%); olanzapine (56%). Although the authors make points to compare groups, the very high rates of sexual dysfunction among all the groups make comparisons of limited clinical meaning. Among the small group of patients (approximately 25%) who did not have sexual problems at baseline, the rates of acquired sexual dysfunction were somewhat lower than for the whole sample. For this group without baseline sexual problems, over the 12 months the onset of new sexual dysfunction, by drug, was as follows: olanzapine, 29%; quetiapine, 34%; risperidone, 43%; haloperidol, 45%. The absence of a placebo comparison group makes assigning drug effects as the cause of sexual function difficult, but it appears that there are minor advantages for olanzapine and quetiapine compared with more potent dopamine antagonists such as haloperidol and risperidone. The authors, unfortunately, did not report what proportion of patients experienced severe sexual dysfunction for each group. For example, if one group had a relatively high rate of severe dysfunction and another group 'some problems', differentiating between groups would be more meaningful.

In a separate analysis examining 570 patients from this same patient sample, investigators reported on sexual functioning in first-time treated patients with schizophrenia at baseline, 3 months and 6 months. Again, in this study funded by the manufacturers of olanzapine, the authors reported that for first-time treated patients, there were advantages for olanzapine compared with risperidone [29]. The advantages, however, were quite small and only statistically significant for libido. For the category 'neuroleptic-related sexual dysfunction' there were no differences between groups after 6 months. Hence, the difference between the two antipsychotics regarding sexual function is likely very small.

Antipsychotics in Bipolar Disorder

Despite the commonplace use of antipsychotics in treating bipolar disorder, there are very few studies evaluating sexual side effects in this population. In one large effectiveness study (n = 329) sponsored by the manufacturer of olanzapine, the authors compared the clinical effects of olanzapine and risperidone in patients with nonpsychotic acute mania [30].

Although the primary aim of the study was to compare antipsychotic effectiveness in controlling mania, tolerability and side effects were also studied. Among the tolerability items, four questions were asked at baseline and at endpoint to measure current sexual interest, ability to become aroused, ability to achieve orgasm, and overall satisfaction. Each item was rated on a 0–4 score, with higher scores indicating worse sexual functioning. At baseline, mean sexual function scores suggested mild to moderate sexual dysfunction. Over the course of the study, total mean sexual scores worsened, though the changes were relatively small. Baseline mean scores for both groups were 7 ± 5 (SD), out of a total of 20, when 20 represent the worse score. At endpoint, the risperidone-treated patients showed mild worsening (mean increase in score of 1.75 points) that was of statistically greater than the mean rise in olanzapine scores (0.65 points). Although the authors highlight this difference in favor of olanzapine, the difference was small and is of questionable clinical relevance.

There are, unfortunately, no studies evaluating sexual dysfunction in bipolar patients treated with antipsychotics along with anticonvulsants or lithium, though the combination of drugs is not likely less than either alone.

Treatment of Antipsychotic-Induced Sexual Dysfunction

There is little systematic study in the treatment of sexual dysfunction associated with antipsychotics. As with antidepressants, the possibilities include selecting a drug with the lowest risk for sexual side effects, dose reduction, switching to a less troublesome drug and using a treatment to reverse the side effect.

At this point, there is no clear evidence that any one of the antipsychotic drugs is superior to the others, though there is a suggestion that the second-generation agents, with the exception of risperidone, may be somewhat less prone to causing sexual side effects than haloperidol. There is, unfortunately no systematic study of ziprasidone or aripiprazole regarding sexual dysfunction. The limited data available suggest that quetiapine or olanzapine may be less problematic than risperidone for causing sexual side effects, but these two drugs are far from being problem free.

Dose reduction makes reasonable sense for any adverse effect, though this method has not been tested, and dose reduction in psychotic disorders risks return of disabling mental illness.

Wafting for tolerance to develop is another possibility, though there is only limited evidence for this approach, and cross-sectional studies suggest that sexual dysfunction may be chronic, though ascribing the problem to the antipsychotic rather than other factors is problematic.

In one 18-week prospective study of 153 young adult inpatients receiving clozapine (n = 100) or haloperidol (n = 53) for schizophrenia, sexual side effects were evaluated weekly for the first 6 weeks and then monthly for 3 months [31]. A person was considered to experience sexual side effects even if the severity was mild. The rater inquired about menstrual changes, desire, erections, orgasm dysfunction, and ejaculatory dysfunction. Side effects were common during the first 6 weeks in both treatment groups. The most common side effect was diminished sexual desire, occurring in approximately 60% of men and 30% of women. Surprisingly, sexual dysfunction was as common in clozapine-treated patients as in haloperidol-treated patients. The severity of the desire problem was not reported. Similarly, erectile dysfunction was also common, but at approximately the same rate (25%) in both patient groups. This finding alone was of interest because it was postulated that clozapine's low affinity for dopamine receptors may have afforded protection against sexual side effects, but clozapine was just as likely to cause erectile dysfunction or loss of desire as haloperidol. More surprisingly, the authors noted that by the end of the study the diminished desire resolved for many of the men (decreased from 53 to 22%) and completely resolved for the women. Additionally, erectile dysfunction and ejaculatory dysfunction 'disappeared within the first 18 weeks of treatment'. These surprising findings have not been replicated, but they suggest that some patients may develop tolerance to antipsychotic-associated sexual dysfunction.

Switching to another drug of less potential to cause sexual side effects is a rational idea, though this method has not been studied adequately and remains, at best, a potential option for further inquiry.

There are no established treatments to reverse antipsychotic-induced sexual dysfunction for women, though limited open-label series and one controlled trial suggests that sildenafil is a well tolerated and effective treatment for erectile dysfunction associated with antipsychotics. In a short-term placebo-controlled crossover study (n = 32), sildenafil, 25–50 mg, was effective for a majority of patients in producing an adequate number erections, satisfaction with sexual intercourse and the duration of erections [32]. In this study, young married men (mean age 35) diagnosed with schizophrenia taking a stable dose of an antipsychotic and erectile dysfunction deemed secondary to an antipsychotic were randomized to sildenafil or placebo for 2 weeks, and then crossed over to the other treatment. Over the course of the study, patients taking sildenafil reported more satisfactory erections (mean 6.5) than placebo-treated patients (mean 3.3). Similarly, more patients treated with sildenafil (77%) reported improvement in erectile functioning compared with placebo-treated patients (23%). Although the improvement in erections and the doubling of number of satisfactory erections is impressive, the time of erections (as determined from a diary) was quite brief in both groups (sildenafil 3.4 min and placebo 2.2 min). There was, unfortunately, no overall satisfaction rating for the sexual experience, though most (74%) patients agreed that they would continue the sildenafil treatment if given the option. Hence, although sildenafil was beneficial, at relatively low doses, the duration of erections was brief. It is possible that doses higher than 50 mg of sildenafil would be of greater value for men with erectile dysfunction associated with schizophrenia. Although this study only evaluated erectile function, it is possible that other facets of sexual function, including interest and frequency may secondarily improve if erectile dysfunction is resolved.

Hence, for antipsychotic-related sexual dysfunction the preliminary evidence is that sildenafil may be effective for reversing erectile dysfunction, at least in healthy young men. It is not known if sildenafil is effective for other groups of patients, including older patients with medical conditions that could affect sexual functioning. There are no treatments established for sexual dysfunction experienced by women treated with antipsychotics.

Antipsychotic Drug Summary

Although there is insufficient study with a placebo control and pretreatment sexual function measures, it appears that the antipsychotics cause sexual dysfunction and that the conditions for which they treat (e.g. schizophrenia) are also associated with sexual dysfunction. All aspects of sexual function are affected, and it is not clear that one aspect is more impaired than another. There are some data, though limited, to suggest that quetiapine and olanzapine may cause fewer sexual side effects than risperidone or first generation antipsychotics, though the evidence is not convincing. Older drugs well known anecdotally to cause sexual dysfunction have not been well studied. The most recent antipsychotics, aripiprazole and ziprasidone, similarly, have not been well studied to ascertain their effects on sexual functioning. Switching antipsychotics has not been shown to be an effective strategy for antipsychotic-associated sexual dysfunction. A preliminary study suggests that sildenafil is a reasonably effective treatment for antipsychotic-associated erectile dysfunction, though more study is needed.

Mood Stabilizers

Lithium

Although there has been extensive study of antidepressant-associated sexual side effects in patients with depressive disorders, there has been very little investigation into patients treated with lithium for bipolar disorder or unipolar depression.

A small open-label study of bipolar and schizoaffective male patients taking lithium as their only medication, found that 31.4% reported sexual dysfunction on a sexual function questionnaire [33]. Patients were all reportedly euthymic at the time of inquiry. Just over 23% of patients reported reduction in frequency of sexual thoughts and 20% of men reported loss of erection during sex. Maintaining erections were reported by 14% of patients. Despite these problems, almost all patients reported normal pleasure during sexual activity and were satisfied with their sexual performance. Serum lithium concentrations were similar between patients with and without sexual dysfunction. Overall, patients reported that sexual dysfunction was minor, did not lead to noncompliance, and was not a source of distress.

A point prevalence evaluation of patients with bipolar disorder found similar results, suggesting that patients treated with lithium as their only medication infrequently experience sexual dysfunction [34]. In this study, 104 patients with bipolar disorder (nearly all of whom were euthymic) were asked to rate the current effects of lithium on sexual functioning 'relative to a period of normal mood when the patient was not taking lithium.' Several parameters of sexual function were rated according to the change affected by lithium, rated as 'none, mild, moderate or great'. The authors found that among patients taking monotherapy lithium, only 14% of patients reported sexual side effects and these were almost all mild. The type of sexual side effect was not detailed for lithium. On the other hand, when lithium was combined with benzodiazepines, rates jumped to 40% of patients, and many of the complaints were moderate or great. This study has a number of limitations, principally that ratings were made retrospectively, sometimes many years after starting lithium. The study had no control group and medication was not randomly assigned. If the benzodiazepines indeed caused sexual problems, it is not clear if they caused them independently of lithium or if in combination with the lithium.

Finally, one recent study, published in Italian, reported that 'clinically stable' patients with bipolar disorder taking lithium were more likely than age-matched healthy controls to report to have 'never' or 'rarely' sexual intercourses (45% vs. 20%), sexual fantasies (25.4 vs. 13.6%), and desire (37.3 vs. 9.5%) [35].

It is unknown from this study how much the patient's mood disorder or medication treatment contributed to their sexual complaints.

Hence, there has been very limited study into the effects of lithium on sexual functioning, though lithium appears to have limited adverse sexual side effects. Further prospective studies are needed.

Anticonvulsants

Little is known about the effects of anticonvulsants on sexual functioning in bipolar patients despite their many years of use. Although there are some reports addressing anticonvulsant effects on sexual function in patients with epilepsy, evaluating this limited information is difficult because sexual dysfunction often accompanies epilepsy. There are a few case reports of ejaculatory failure related to carbamazepine and gabapentin, but the frequency of this possible effect is unknown. Little is known about sexual side effects of the commonly used anticonvulsant, divalproex. At best there are a few case reports suggesting that divalproex may reduce libido or the ability to achieve orgasm in women, though there are no prospective controlled studies to delineate the extent of this possible problem. There is a suggestion that lamotrigine may have some advantages over the other anticonvulsants regarding sexual side effects, but this is preliminary.

In one study of 62 patients, women and men showed modest overall improvement in sexual function scores when switched from another anticonvulsant to lamotrigine [36]. Because of the lack of control group and the possible confound of epilepsy of sexual function, it is difficult to extend these findings to patients with mood disorders, though it suggests that lamotrigine may have fewer sexual side effects than other anticonvulsants.

Phenytoin and carbamazepine induce metabolism of androgens, while divalproex inhibits this metabolism. This would suggest that phenytoin and carbamazepine could be problem prone and valproate less problem prone, though prospective study is lacking. Valproic acid has not been studied prospectively in samples of patients with bipolar disorder for its effects on androgens and sexual functioning. There are, however, several case reports of reduced libido or orgasm inability in patients with mood disorders treated with divalproex [37].

A cross-sectional, nonrandomized study of 75 men with epilepsy found that sexual dysfunction was more commonly associated with phenytoin (n = 25) and carbamazepine (n = 25) than with control patients (n = 25) or lamotrigine (n = 25) treated patients [38]. Lamotrigine-treated patients reported sexual symptoms at approximately the same rate as a normal control group. In this study, patients rated sexual functioning on a rating scale that measured 'sexual interest and potency' as well as had blood measured for gonadal hormones, including luteinizing hormone, follicle-stimulating hormone, prolactin, testosterone and estradiol. Mean sexual function scores for lamotrigine were slightly higher, and statistically greater compared with the carbamazepine and phenytoin groups. The effect size, however, was quite small. Additionally, testosterone concentrations were lower in the carbamazepine- and phenytoin-treated patients compared with the lamotrigine treated patients, which were similar to controls. Although this information may not be extended to patients without epilepsy, it appears that lamotrigine is less prone toward causing sexual dysfunction than carbamazepine and phenytoin, though none of the anticonvulsants may seriously affect sexual functioning.

Anxiolytic Drugs

Benzodiazepines

The benzodiazepines have not been prospectively studied regarding their effects on sexual function. There are a number of retrospective reports suggesting that clonzepam may be problematic for sexual functioning, though other reports suggest that it might not be problematic. All of the benzodiazepines have been suggested to cause sexual dysfunction, but there are no prospective studies examining sexual function in patients taking this class of medication for an anxiety disorder. Considering the frequency of their use, the lack of reports suggests that the side effects may be of minor importance. Moreover, without baseline measure before drug initiation, some of the reported sexual dysfunction may be related to the mood or anxiety disorders for which they are prescribed. The few reports available for review are cross-sectional or retrospective in small samples and rating scales were not necessarily employed. Decreases in libido, arousal, and orgasm have all been reported. In one study, detailed in the 'Lithium' section above, the authors found that benzodiazepines combined with lithium in the treatment of bipolar disorder patients caused 40% of patients to experience sexual side effects, which was considerably higher than the 14% rate in patients taking only lithium. The study did not evaluate if the effects were specifically associated with arousal, orgasm or libido for the combination of lithium and benzodiazepines. On the other hand, an early small placebo-controlled study in normal patients without anxiety found that diazepam 'facilitated sexual behaviors in normals' [39].

While some sexual dysfunction in patients with anxiety disorders taking benzodiazepines may be attributable to benzodiazepines, the effects of benzodiazepines on sexual function clearly need further prospective study to determine the extent and clinical relevance.

Buspirone

Buspirone is an anxiolytic that does not appear to have sexual side effects, though it has not been specifically studied in prospective studies for its propensity to cause sexual side effects. Interestingly, as noted in the antidepressant section, buspirone may reverse sexual dysfunction associated with serotonin reuptake antidepressant use. It appears that this benefit is only with relatively high doses, approximately 45–60 mg per day. Without further study, it remains unknown if buspirone monotherapy causes any adverse or salutary sexual effects.

Conclusion

Many psychotropics and mental disorders are associated with sexual dysfunction, though the exact magnitude and phase of sexual functioning affected remains to be elucidated for most psychotropic drugs. Although all phases of sexual functioning may be impaired by psychotropics, SSRI antidepressants appear to primarily affect orgasm, while antipsychotics primarily affect desire. None of the SSRI antidepressants or second-generation antipsychotics stands out as clearly superior to the others in their drug class. Sexual dysfunction appears common in patients with depressive and psychotic disorders, though it is unclear how much of the sexual trouble is due to the illness and how much to the medication. Little has been studied regarding sexual function in patients with multiple psychotropic medications or medical conditions. Much less is known about the mood stabilizers or anxiolytics and how they affect sexual functioning, though these classes of medication appear somewhat less problem prone. Evaluating sexual function before and after starting psychotropics remains an important clinical and research agenda. Limited treatments are available for the treatment of sexual dysfunction, though sildenafil appears moderately effective for antidepressant- or antipsychotic-induced erectile dysfunction.

References

1. Casper RC, Redmond DE Jr, Katz MM, Schaffer CB, Davis JM, Koslow SH: Somatic symptoms in primary affective disorder. Presence and relationship to the classification of depression. Arch Gen Psychiatry 1985;42:1098–1104.
2. Montejo-González AL, Llorca G, Izquierdo JA, Ledesma A, Bousoño M, Calcedo A, Carrasco JL, Ciudad J, Daniel E, De la Gandara J, Derecho J, Franco M, Gomez MJ, Macias JA, Martin T, Perez V, Sanchez JM, Sanchez S, Vicens EJ: SSSRI-induced sexual dysfunction: fluoxetine, paroxetine, sertraline, and fluvoxamine in a prospective, multicenter, and descriptive clinical study of 344 patients. Sex Marital Ther 1997;23:176–194.
3. Landén M, Högberg P: Thase ME: Incidence of sexual side effects in refractory depression during treatment with citalopram or paroxetine.J Clin Psychiatry 2005;66:100–106.
4. Nicolosi A, Laumann EO, Glasser DB, Moreira ED Jr, Paik A, Gingell C: Global Study of Sexual Attitudes and Behaviors Investigators' Group: Sexual behavior and sexual dysfunctions after age 40: the global study of sexual attitudes and behaviors. Urol 2004;64:991–997.
5. Thase ME, Clayton AH, Haight BR, Thompson AH, Modell JG, Johnston JA: A double-blind comparison between bupropion XL and venlafaxine XR: sexual functioning, antidepressant efficacy, and tolerability. J Clin Psychopharmacol 2006;26:482–488.
6. Behnke K, Søgaard J, Martin S, Bäuml J, Ravindran AV, Agren H, Vester-Blokland ED: Mirtazapine orally disintegrating tablet versus sertraline: a prospective onset of action study. J Clin Psychopharmacol 2003; 23:358–364.

7 Coleman CC, King BR, Bolden-Watson C, Book MJ, Segraves RT, Richard N, Ascher J, Batey S, Jamerson B, Metz A: A placebo-controlled comparison of the effects on sexual functioning of bupropion sustained release and fluoxetine. Clin Ther 2001;23:1040–1058.

8 Segraves RT, Kavoussi R, Hughes AR, Batey SR, Johnston JA, Donahue R, Ascher JA: Evaluation of sexual functioning in depressed outpatients: a double-blind comparison of sustained-release bupropion and sertraline treatment. J Clin Psychopharmacol 2000;20:122–128.

9 Clayton AH, Zajecka J, Ferguson JM, Filipiak-Reisner JK, Brown MT, Schwartz GE: Lack of sexual dysfunction with the selective noradrenaline reuptake inhibitor reboxetine during treatment for major depressive disorder. Int Clin Psychopharmacol 2003; 18:151–156.

10 Delgado PL, Brannan SK, Mallinckrodt CH, Tran PV, McNamara RK, Wang F, Watkin JG, Detke MJ: Sexual functioning assessed in 4 double-blind placebo- and paroxetine-controlled trials of duloxetine for major depressive disorder. J Clin Psychiatry 2005;66:686–692.

11 Montejo AL, Llorca G, Izquierdo JA, Rico-Villademoros F: Spanish Working Group for the Study of Psychotropic-Related Sexual Dysfunction: Incidence of sexual dysfunction associated with antidepressant agents: a prospective multicenter study of 1022 outpatients. J Clin Psychiatry 2001;62 (suppl 3):10–21.

12 Waldinger MD, Zwinderman AH, Olivier B: Antidepressants and ejaculation: a double-blind, randomized, fixed-dose study with mirtazapine and paroxetine. J Clin Psychopharmacol 2003;23: 467–470.

13 Gelenberg AJ, McGahuey C, Laukes C, Okayli G, Moreno F, Zentner L, Delgado P: Mirtazapine substitution in SSSRI-induced sexual dysfunction. J Clin Psychiatry 2000;61:356–360.

14 Ferguson JM, Shrivastava RK, Stahl SM, Hartford JT, Borian F, Ieni J, McQuade RD, Jody DJ: Reemergence of sexual dysfunction in patients with major depressive disorder: double-blind comparison of nefazodone and sertraline. Clin Psychiatry 2001;62:24–29.

15 Labbate LA, Grimes JB, Hines A, Pollack MH: Bupropion treatment of serotonin reuptake antidepressant-associated sexual dysfunction. Ann Clin Psychiatry 1997;9:241–245.

16 Clayton AH, Warnock JK, Kornstein SG, Pinkerton R, Sheldon-Keller A, McGarvey EL: A placebo-controlled trial of bupropion SR as an antidote for selective serotonin reuptake inhibitor-induced sexual dysfunction. J Clin Psychiatry 2004;65:62–67.

17 Landén M, Eriksson E, Agren H, Fahlén T: Effect of buspirone on sexual dysfunction in depressed patients treated with selective serotonin reuptake inhibitors. J Clin Psychopharmacol 1999;19:268–271.

18 Seidman SN, Roose SP, Menza MA, Shabsigh R, Rosen RC: Treatment of erectile dysfunction in men with depressive symptoms: results of a placebo-controlled trial with sildenafil citrate. Am J Psychiatry 2001;158:1623–1630.

19 Fava M, Nurnberg HG, Seidman SN, Holloway W, Nicholas S, Tseng LJ, Stecher VJ: Efficacy and safety of sildenafil in men with serotonergic antidepressant-associated erectile dysfunction: results from a randomized, double-blind, placebo-controlled trial. J Clin Psychiatry 2006;67:240–246.

20 Nurnberg HG, Hensley PL, Gelenberg AJ, Fava M, Lauriello J, Paine S: Treatment of antidepressant-associated sexual dysfunction with sildenafil: a randomized controlled trial. JAMA 2003;289:56–64.

21 Dossenbach M, Hodge A, Anders M, Molnár B, Peciukaitiene D, Krupka-Matuszczyk I, Tatu M, Bondar V, Pecenak J, Gorjanc T, McBride M: Prevalence of sexual dysfunction in patients with schizophrenia: international variation and underestimation. Int J Neuropsychopharmacol 2005;8:195–201.

22 Kelly DL, Conley RR: A randomized double-blind 12-week study of quetiapine, risperidone or fluphenazine on sexual functioning in people with schizophrenia. Psychoneuroendocrinology 2006;31:340–346.

23 Knegtering H, Boks M, Blijd C, Castelein S, van den Bosch RJ, Wiersma D: A randomized open-label comparison of the impact of olanzapine versus risperidone on sexual functioning. J Sex Marital Ther 2006;32:315–326.

24 Nakonezny PA, Byerly MJ, Rush AJ: The relationship between serum prolactin level and sexual functioning among male outpatients with schizophrenia or schizoaffective disorder: a randomized double-blind trial of risperidone vs. quetiapine. J Sex Marital Ther 2007;33:203–216.

25 Bobes J, Garc A-Portilla MP, Rejas J, Hern Ndez G, Garcia-Garcia M, Rico-Villademoros F, Porras A: Frequency of sexual dysfunction and other reproductive side-effects in patients with schizophrenia treated with risperidone, olanzapine, quetiapine, or haloperidol: the results of the EIRE study. J Sex Marital Ther 2003;29:125–147.

26 Uçok A, Incesu C, Aker T, Erkoç S: Sexual dysfunction in patients with schizophrenia on antipsychotic medication. Eur Psychiatry 2007;22:328–333.

27 Byerly MJ, Nakonezny PA, Bettcher BM, Carmody T, Fisher R, Rush AJ: Sexual dysfunction associated with second-generation antipsychotics in outpatients with schizophrenia or schizoaffective disorder: an empirical evaluation of olanzapine, risperidone, and quetiapine. Schizophr Res 2006;86:244–250.

28 Dossenbach M, Dyachkova Y, Pirildar S, Anders M, Khalil A, Araszkiewicz A, Shakhnovich T, Akram A, Pecenak J, McBride M, Treuer T: Effects of atypical and typical antipsychotic treatments on sexual function in patients with schizophrenia: 12-month results from the Intercontinental Schizophrenia Outpatient Health Outcomes (IC-SOHO) study. Eur Psychiatry 2006;21:251–258.

29 Bitter I, Basson BR, Dossenbach MR: Antipsychotic treatment and sexual functioning in first-time neuroleptic-treated schizophrenic patients. Int Clin Psychopharmacol 2005;20:19–21.

30 Perlis RH, Baker RW, Zarate CA Jr, Brown EB, Schuh LM, Jamal HH, Tohen M: Olanzapine versus risperidone in the treatment of manic or mixed States in bipolar I disorder: a randomized, double-blind trial. J Clin Psychiatry 2006;67:1747–1753.

31 Hummer M, Kemmler G, Kurz M, Kurzthaler I, Oberbauer H, Fleischhacker WW: Sexual disturbances during clozapine and haloperidol treatment for schizophrenia. Am J Psychiatry 1999;156: 631–633.

32 Gopalakrishnan R, Jacob KS, Kuruvilla A, Vasantharaj B, John JK: Sildenafil in the treatment of antipsychotic-induced erectile dysfunction: a randomized, double-blind, placebo-controlled, flexible-dose, two-way crossover trial. Am J Psychiatry 2006;163:494–499.

33 Aizenberg D, Sigler M, Zemishlany Z, Weizman A: Lithium and male sexual function in affective patients. Clin Neuropharmacol 1996;19:515–519.

34 Ghadirian AM, Annable L, Bélanger MC: Lithium, benzodiazepines, and sexual function in bipolar patients. Am J Psychiatry 1992;149:801–805.

35 Zuncheddu C, Carpiniello B: Sexual dysfunctions and bipolar disorder: a study of patients submitted to a long- term lithium treatment Clin Ter 2006;157: 419–424.

36 Gil-Nagel A, López-Muñoz F, Serratosa JM, Moncada I, García-García P, Alamo C: Effect of lamotrigine on sexual function in patients with epilepsy Seizure 2006;15:142–149.

37 Schneck CD, Thomas MR, Gundersen D: Sexual side effects associated with valproate. J Clin Psychopharmacol 2002;22:532–534.

38 Herzog AG, Drislane FW, Schomer DL, Pennell PB, Bromfield EB, Dworetzky BA, Farina EL, Frye CA: Differential effects of antiepileptic drugs on sexual function and hormones in men with epilepsy. Neurology 2005 11;65:980–981.

39 Dasberg HH: Effects and plasma levels of N-desmethyldiazepam after oral administration in normal volunteers. Psychopharmacologia 1975;43: 191–198.

Lawrence A. Labbate, MD
Department of Psychiatry, University of Arkansas for Medical Sciences
4301 W Markham Street
Little Rock, AR 72205 (USA)
Tel. +1 501 686 5900, Fax +1 501 257 3164, E-Mail llabbate@uams.edu

Balon R (ed): Sexual Dysfunction. The Brain-Body Connection.
Adv Psychosom Med. Basel, Karger, 2008, vol 29, pp 131–149

Drugs of Abuse and Sexual Functioning

António Pacheco Palha · Manuel Esteves

Department of Psychiatry, Oporto Medical School, Porto, Portugal

Abstract

The use of mind-altering substances can be found in very different cultures and traced back thousands of years; the same is true for the searching of drugs that could increase sexual functioning. In this text, we explore the relation between drugs of abuse and sexuality in three domains: drugs and sexual dysfunctions, drugs and risky sexual behavior and drugs used as sexual aids. Although some drugs can increase sexual response in the early stages of the addiction career, particularly in those with a previous sexual dysfunction, the chronic use of substances tends to deteriorate all stages of sexual response in both male and female abusers. There is sufficient evidence for considering that drug use before or during sexual intercourse can, in certain circumstances, elevate the risk of unwanted pregnancy or sexually transmitted diseases. Specific prevention strategies should be addressed to this population. Some psychotropic drugs are sometimes used as sexual aids. This can have some risks and should alert the therapist to a possible underlying and undiagnosed sexual problem.

Perhaps the first relation between drugs and sexual functioning was the desire to increase sexual performance by the use of a substance.

Aphrodisiacs were thus agents believed to increase sexual desire and derived its name from Aphrodite, the Greek goddess of love, beauty and sexual rapture.

The search for such substances dates back millennia. Aphrodisiacs can be classified by their alleged action in those that would increase libido, potency or sexual pleasure [1].

A variety of food, drinks and animal and vegetal derivatives has been used for this purpose by folk medicines of different cultures. Sometimes those beliefs were based on the principles of *sympathetic magic* ('likes produce likes'). According to this, and due to its shape, the horn of a rhinoceros would increase male sexuality or oysters, female sexuality. In some cultures, aphrodisiacs for increasing virility were obtained from the tiger penis.

Other substances such as ambrein, constituent of *Ambra grisea* used in Arab countries, cantharidin ('spanish fly'), bufo toad skin and glans used in preparations in the West Indians and China and the *Panax ginseng* also used in China may have some pharmacological properties that would explain their use for centuries [1].

With the scientific study of medicinal agents and the advent of pharmacology, the use of these substances was progressively dismissed. According to Nordenberg [2], the Food and Drug Administration found that the reputed sexual effects of those aphrodisiacs are based upon folklore rather than scientific facts.

We must, however, not overlook the importance of the placebo effect. As the enjoyment of all the senses and the human capacity for imagination and fantasy lie at the bases of sexual stimulation, some people may find some perfumes, aromatic oils, beverages or foods particularly stimulating [3].

With the increasing number of new pharmaceutical drugs, it became obvious that some of them had positive and some negative effects on sexual functioning. The interest in the study of alcohol and drug abuse made also obvious the effect of these substances on sexual response.

This text will focus on the effects exerted by drugs of abuse on the sexuality of their users.

Sex and Drugs

The relation of drug abuse and sexuality has been studied in its several interactions, namely, sexual dysfunctions linked to the use of drugs [4], the use of drugs and risk of sexually transmitted diseases (STDs) [5], and the use of drugs to improve sexual performance [6, 7].

It seems reasonable to assume that lower doses of substances will have different impact on sexuality than higher doses, and it has been established, as we will see later, that the acute use of a drug can have very different consequences on sexuality than chronic drug use.

Drugs and Sexual/Marital Relationship

Drug users may experience sexuality differently from healthy populations. They may acquire painful and distorted ideas about sexuality. Checcucci [8] found that many young addicted people included in her therapeutic group were apprehensive about participating, because they had recollections of failure, violence, prostitution and hidden anxiety, that they had never allowed to emerge and had been internalized as something dirty and never to be shared with others. Drug addicts may even use violent forms of sexuality for hiding fear or a sense of inadequacy or inferiority, for which they do not find a healthy way to cope. The addiction career can produce forms of sexual behavior felt as degrading, such as prostitution (even among males).

Although not specific to drug addicts, they tend to acquire their sexual information in a distorted way, mainly from their peers [8]. But in drug addicts, the lack of adequate sexual information appears to be linked to a general lack of education. Premature dropout from school and dysfunctional families of origin may have an influence on poor sex education.

The same author [8] also found that the sexuality of the drug user appears to be influenced by several stereotypes (not specific to addicts) based in the male culture and the urge to transgress. Precocious sexual behavior and the desire to have experiences seem to be part of a search for sensations.

The lifestyle of the typical addict is not really consistent with a durable or healthy affective or sexual relationship.

Drug addicts may lack the social skills to engage in an affective/sexual relationship and when involved in one, the relationships tend to be considered unhappy [9]. The attention almost always focused on drugs, the reduced or dysfunctional sexuality and the lack of other nondrug activities seriously undermine the relationship [10]. Arguments about drugs and money are frequent, and when just one in the couple is an addict suspicion and secrecy are factors of important stress for the couple.

Drugs and Sexual Dysfunctions

Drug abusers frequently experience sexual dysfunctions sometimes previously to their addiction, and sometimes as a result of their habit. In any case, these sexual problems can perpetuate dependence or constitute a therapeutic tool, seldom used by addiction therapists.

When the sex life of drug users is studied, almost all components of sexual response can be found impaired. This is particularly true if we direct our attention to the dependent patient with a chronic and frequent use of drugs.

Alcohol

Alcohol has been used as an aphrodisiac for millennia, mainly due to its disinhibition properties. The consumption of alcohol often precedes sexual activity and it is commonly believed that alcohol is a powerful sexual facilitator and aphrodisiac [11]. While alcohol consumption can indeed act as a disinhibitor, leading some people to be more receptive to sexual activity, the belief that alcohol can intensify sexual response is a myth. Indeed, alcohol typically has the opposite effect, particularly in large quantities, impairing the sexual response.

The acute effects of its ingestion may interfere with erection, vaginal lubrication and orgasm. These effects have also been known for centuries, their most famous historical description being that of Shakespeare in Macbeth (act II, scene III) – 'It provoketh desire and taketh away the capacity'. Nevertheless, the retardant effect over the orgasm may be appreciated by some men with a tendency to ejaculate precociously; however, this effect will be undesired in those men and women with orgasm difficulties [7]. In the alcoholics, a number of sexual dysfunctions can be observed ranging from desire inhibition, arousal and orgasmic difficulties to menstrual problems and infertility. In men, a process of feminization can be observed.

The mechanisms behind these dysfunctions can be related to the alcohol-induced hepatic catabolism of testosterone and its conversion, mediated by the enzyme aromatase, in estradiol [12, 13]. Feminization associated with chronic alcohol intake in men has also been attributed to the phytoestrogen content of alcoholic beverages [14, 15].

Alcohol inhibits the hypothalamic-pituitary-adrenal axis traduced in low levels of gonadotropin-releasing factor, gonadotropin, luteinizing hormone and follicle stimulant hormone, also lowering sex hormones (testosterone, estradiol and progesterone) at the gonad level. The chronic abuse of alcohol may cause testicular atrophy, inhibition of testosterone production and inhibition of spermatogenesis, apart from its direct oxidative toxicity [16, 17]. Spermatozoid number, morphology and mobility can be significantly altered in these patients.

As a result of reduction in estradiol levels, women with chronic alcohol abuse may present impaired vaginal lubrication and dyspareunia. Hyperprolactinemia with menstrual irregularities or amenorrhea can also be present.

Prolonged alcohol intake may lead to loss of vasopressin and oxytocin neurons in the hypothalamus [18]. It is known that oxytocin is a hormone released during the sexual response and has been linked to the increase of this response and the arousal in women [19, 20].

Tobacco

There is abundant experimental research on the interference of tobacco smoking and sexual function, particularly in male sexuality [21, 22].

In a revision of literature, Dorey [23] concluded that male smokers have a 1.5 greater probability of developing erectile dysfunction than nonsmokers. This risk appears to be associated with the intensity of the addiction correlating with the number of cigarettes smoked per day and the number of years of smoking habit [24]. The impact of smoking on erectile function, although more evident in older men, can be found in men under the age of 45 years [25].

The impact of smoking on sexual function can be easily explained if we consider that nicotine is a potent vasoconstrictor. The physical components of the arousal phase (i.e. erection in the male, swelling of the clitoris and genital engorgement in the female) requires efficient blood flow to the genital area and nicotine reduces the efficiency of blood circulation to these areas. In men, smoking contributes to vasculogenic erectile dysfunction because of the effects of smoke on the vascular endothelium and peripheral nerves. In addition, blood nicotine levels rise after smoking, and this may increase the sympathetic tone in the penis, via nicotine-induced smooth muscle contraction interfering with corporal smooth muscle relaxation needed to produce and maintain an erection [26]. Wolf and Shulman [27] in their review of the etiology of nicotine-related sexual dysfunction consider that endothelium-derived relaxing factor, nitric oxide, prostaglandin, prostacycline and thromboxane changes may contribute to smoking-induced impotence. Studies concerning the endocrine profile showed elevated serum levels of estradiol in smokers. The results of testosterone levels are contradictory.

Of smokers, 86% have an abnormal penile vascular evaluation and ultrastructural damage has been detected in corporal tissue of men with erectile dysfunction who are chronic smokers [26].

A decrease of 13–17% in sperm density is observed in smokers when compared with nonsmokers. Although this does not constitute a risk factor for difficult conception, it can be an important issue in men with marginal semen quality or other risk factors [27].

Cigarette smoking, apart from being clearly linked to a higher risk of erectile dysfunction, also has an immediate negative impact on a man's ability to get and maintain a strong erection [11].

While there has been no research on the direct impact of smoking on female sexual function, it is clear that smoking reduces blood flow to the lower extremities, and to the extent that female sexual arousal involves blood flow to the genital area, it is logical to speculate that cigarette smoking may inhibit physical sexual arousal among women [11].

Not smoking, even for short periods of time, can improve sexual function. In addition, there is evidence that quitting smoking can have a longer-term benefit on sexual function [11, 28].

Cannabis

The use of cannabis has a history of many centuries [29] and through time has been associated with sexual behavior.

There has been no direct scientific investigation of the impact of cannabis consumption on the physiological components of the sexual response cycle [11].

Research, conducted with marijuana smokers, suggests that many users perceive that it has a beneficial impact. In the most extensive study of the sexual effects of regular marijuana smoking, 76% of female users and 70% of male users reported that marijuana increased sexual pleasure and satisfaction and 58% of males and 36% of females reported that smoking marijuana enhanced the orgasm quality [30]. Most marijuana users in this study also reported that it had mild aphrodisiac effects.

The principal positive effect, regarding sexuality, seems to be associated with the disinhibition provided by Δ-9-THC, its main active component. In fact it seems to favor relaxation in the physical contact with the partner, to stimulate erotic fantasies, to alter the space and time perception and to reduce aggression [7].

It has also been suggested that the enhancement of sexual experiences from marijuana use can be modulated by the expectations of users, personality type, age, consumption setting, and relationship status of the couple [31].

Perceived positive effects are less likely to occur when increasing amounts of the drug are consumed [11]. Although high enough doses of THC may inhibit the hypothalamic-pituitary-adrenal axis, the studies searching a relevant hormonal effect remain contradictory according to the revision by Saso [7].

The impact of long-term marijuana use on sexuality and sexual function is unclear as the very limited research on this topic has produced apparently conflicting results [11].

Opioids

In the initial stages of opioid abuse, some patients experience an improvement in sexual function. In women, this has been related to the relaxation induced by opiate substances and to their analgesic effect in cases of dyspareunia and vaginismus. In men, drug-induced delay of orgasm may be valued by those who experienced rapid ejaculation prior to drug abuse [32]. As dependence grows and drug use becomes a daily routine, women may report anorgasmia and amenorrhea; men may report decrease libido, erectile dysfunction and delayed ejaculation.

Opioid abusers entering outpatient therapy were studied by King et al. [33]. 95% of subjects reported being sexually active during the past year, and the median number of sexual partners was 1. Rates of monogamy, sexual abstinence and condom use were comparable to rates in the general population. 15.8% reported some involvement in commercial sexual activity; these subjects reported higher rates of condom use. Few subjects however used condoms with any consistency.

In regular users, decreased libido has been found in the majority of addicts, erectile dysfunction in 39–48% and delayed ejaculation in over 50% of addicts [34–36].

In our own study [37] of a population of 101 heroin addicts compared with a control group of matched healthy subjects, we found a significant decrease in weekly sexual intercourse and masturbatory activity in men, but not in women. 75% of men and 68% of women felt that heroin decreased their interest in sex (although 5% of men and 20% of women stated an increase in libido). Similarly, 71% of men and 60% of women felt that drug use worsened their sexual arousal (5% of men and 18% of women reported increased arousal). Approximately 60% of the addicts of both sexes felt that drug use decreased their ability to experience orgasm (8% of men and 15% of women stated increase in the ability to experience orgasm). When questioned about the first 6 months of heroin use 21% of men and 28% of women felt their sexual satisfaction had increased. All men with previous premature ejaculation stated that orgasm had improved since the use of heroin.

As we just observed, some men may appreciate the orgasm-retardant properties of opioids, and some women may appreciate the effect on anxiety or pain related to sexual intercourse, mainly during the first phases of opioid use. Others may find it useful in situations of sexual repression or sex aversion [7].

There appears to be a biological basis for the loss of desire and other sexual difficulties related to opioid use.

Although not entirely clear, the underlying mechanism may be the inhibition of the hypothalamic-pituitary-gonadal axis and the increase in prolactin levels. Heroin exerts a depletion effect on plasma levels of free testosterone and raises testosterone-binding globulin levels, irrespective of age, amount of heroin intake per day and period of contact with the drug. Luteinizing hormone, follicle stimulant hormone levels and the response to LHRH are unaffected, suggesting that chronic heroin abuse depresses testicular function via the hypothalamus or higher centers. These hormonal changes returned promptly to normal after withdrawal [38–41].

The same decrease in testosterone levels can be found in methadone-treated patients [42], and the same sexual difficulties described can be observed. These dysfunctions can be troublesome enough for the patient to abandon treatment [7].

Acute administration of heroin seems to produce an intense feeling of pleasure akin to orgasm ('pharmacogenic orgasm') [43, 44]. Heroin may become to its users the 'only great love', a kind of 'good mother', who is able to take them in, console them, reduce the pain and help them to survive [8].

The above observations can have their biological explanation in the action of opiates (and other drugs) on the mesolimbic dopamine reward pathway. This system is intended to organize behavior towards goals that are beneficial to the individual or the species. Some drugs quickly and uniformly exert extreme control over behavior (e.g. heroin, cocaine) with deterioration in the ability of normal rewards (including sex) to govern behavior (effect termed *motivational toxicity*) [45].

Hypersexuality episodes may be observed in men experiencing opiate withdrawal, with spontaneous erections and nocturnal ejaculations [32, 46]. Premature ejaculation may also be observed as a symptom of the withdrawal syndrome or reflecting the pattern previous to the addiction [32, 35, 47].

The unwanted sexual effects of opiates lead to the hypothesis of using opiate antagonists (naloxone and naltrexone) in some erectile dysfunctions, with inconclusive results [48, 49].

Concomitant psychopathology may contribute to some extent in drug-related sexual dysfunction. In their study about comorbidity in heroin addicts, Palha and Esteves [50] found that sexual problems were more prevalent among depressed patients and raised the hypothesis of depression as a contributor to sexual dysfunction among heroin users.

Cocaine

Cocaine does not directly or specifically impact on the human sexual response cycle. However, like for other nervous system stimulants, the feelings of well being that result from taking the drug may intensify or enhance feelings of sexual desire and sensuality [11].

Cocaine appears to have two opposite effects on sexuality according to its acute or chronic abuse. Due to its dopaminergic effects desire and arousal can be augmented, but orgasm tends to be inhibited, which can be appreciated by men with a precocious ejaculation pattern, but can be fastidious in others. For women, this delayed orgasm is undesired [7].

In this way, new or infrequent cocaine users may report that cocaine has beneficial sexual effects, most notably in increasing desire [51].

Regular and long-term use of cocaine, snorted, injected, or smoked (crack) has significant negative effects on sexual functioning, apart from the overall health of the user. Cocaine use increases the individual's risk for a variety of cardiovascular conditions and has been found to be associated with permanent reduced cognitive functioning and with increased risk for delayed mental/cognitive development in infants whose mothers used cocaine during pregnancy [11].

MacDonald et al. [52] in a study of regular cocaine users found that this use was associated with erection difficulties in 66% of men who had been using the drug for 1 year or longer. As for crack cocaine, Wetherby et al. [53] found a negative impact on desire in 57% of subjects and in 63% a decreased ability to reach orgasm, although 37% stated that the drug increased desire and 24% noted a benefit in orgasm.

New users of cocaine may perceive a sexual benefit from taking the drug, and this effect is likely the result of the overall feelings of well-being, confidence, and energy that are associated with the drug. However, it is clear that the regular use of cocaine is not only detrimental to various aspects of physical and mental health, but it can negatively impact on the desire, arousal, and orgasm phases of the sexual response cycle.

The study by Henderson et al. [54] describing the sexual feelings and sexual function of 100 African-American women using large amounts of crack cocaine, did not support the commonly held notion that crack is an aphrodisiac for women and that crack makes women want sex. Furthermore, the women in this study had a higher level of sexual dysfunction.

With chronic abuse of cocaine, sexual dysfunction is attributed mainly to hyperprolactinemia and *downregulation* of the hypothalamic dopaminergic receptors [7].

There are reports of cases of priapism associated with intracavernosal injection of cocaine [55].

Amphetamines

Methamphetamine is a highly addictive drug. Long-term use is associated with increased risk for serious cardiovascular and lung disease, depression, psychosis and cognitive impairment [56].

Over the years, amphetamines have gained the reputation of being able to increase sexual desire, extend the sexual relation and making orgasm more intense. Animal studies showed facilitated sexual behavior in rats injected with D-amphetamine [57]. However, human observational studies revealed a variety of amphetamine-related sexual dysfunctions [58].

These variations may depend on a number of factors: dosage, route of administration, habits of the drug user and social setting. Low doses can increase enjoyment and lower inhibitions. The delayed orgasm may be appreciated by men with rapid ejaculation. With high doses, people of both sexes fail to achieve orgasm and become disinterested in sex. When the drug is injected, some people experience intense 'highs', sexual desire lowers, and physical contact decreases dramatically [59].

Many users of this drug report that methamphetamine acts as an aphrodisiac, reduces sexual inhibitions, and increases satisfaction [60]. Among the so-called 'club drugs' or 'party drugs', methamphetamine is the most strongly associated with sexuality and sexual behavior [11]. This appears to be due to the combination of increased social confidence, sexual disinhibition, and heightened sense of physical energy, perceived as sexual enhancement effects by its users [61].

Methamphetamine does not act directly in any of the specific aspects of the sexual response cycle. But being a powerful nervous system stimulant, it enhances a person's general sense of well-being and excitement which, as a result, is likely to intensify and enhance sexual experiences [11].

For many people, sex under the influence of methamphetamine rapidly leads to an incredibly strong association between the two which is hard to break. One without the other becomes inconceivable [11].

Prolonged use of amphetamine-based drugs has been associated with erectile dysfunction and delayed ejaculation in men as well as delayed orgasm in women [51]. In addition, prolonged use of methamphetamine is strongly associated with a condition called 'crystal dick' in which the user maintains a strong libido, has high energy and lowered sexual inhibitions, but is unable to get an erection [63].

An assessment of the impact of methamphetamine on sexuality must take into account the fact that this drug increases the likelihood for gay, bisexual, and heterosexual methamphetamine users to engage in very high HIV/STI sexual risk behaviors [60, 62, 53].

There have been reports of amphetamine users participating in sexual activities they did not usually practice when they were drug free [59]. A strong association has been found between consumption of the drug and increases in unsafe sexual behavior that places methamphetamine users at high risk for HIV and other STDs [64]. This association may be explained by, among others, the combination of lowered sexual inhibitions, high libido and energy, and the highly charged sexual context in which methamphetamine use often takes place [11].

When compared with intravenous narcotics users, oral users of amphetamines were found to have less disruption of sexual functioning [58].

Ecstasy

Ecstasy (3,4 methylenedioxymethamphetamine or MDMA) is structurally related to the stimulant amphetamine and the hallucinogen mescaline and believed by many to be a 'love drug'. Its acute effects appear to be mediated by the release and reuptake inhibition of serotonin and dopamine [65]. Dopamine has been implicated as facilitator and serotonin as an inhibitor of sexual function [66].

Zemishlany et al. [67] studied the subjective effects of MDMA on human sexual function. All subjects reported an increased sexual desire after MDMA use. The sexual experience was described by most subjects as more sensual than usual. Similarly, 90% of the males and 93% of the females reported an increase in satisfaction. Equivocal responses were obtained with regarding erection: 40% of the males reported a negative effect and 40% a positive effect. In women, 80% reported that lubrication was enhanced. Delay in achieving orgasm while under the influence of MDMA was reported by 80% of the males and 40% of the females. Although the orgasm was delayed in many users, it was perceived to be more intense in 85% of the men and 53% of the women.

These results are in line with the San Francisco study [68] where subjects reported that MDMA enhanced sensuality, made orgasm more difficult to achieve, and decreased erectile ability in 46% of the males.

The activation of the dopaminergic system by MDMA may account for the increase in desire and satisfaction. The inhibitory effect on orgasm is similar to that induced by the selective serotonin reuptake inhibitors, and may be related to stimulation of the serotonergic system [67]. The same authors suggest that some of the self-reported changes in sexual functioning might be due to expected effects of the substance ('placebo effect').

Cases of priapism related to the use of ecstasy have been described [69].

Polydrug Abuse

It is also important to consider polyuse of drugs with possibly unexpected and reciprocal interactions and the association of illicit drugs with benzodiazepines. Benzodiazepines cause drowsiness, thus reducing desire, although in certain doses they can be disinhibitors and may increase libido [4].

Date Rape Drugs

In the last few years, lay and scientific press has raised the awareness of the involvement of licit and illicit drugs in the crime of 'date rape'. The term 'date rape drug' has been coined and has been used to label a few specific drugs because of their alleged properties [70]. These include flunitrazepam, gamma hydroxybutyrate (GHB) and ketamine.

The surreptitious administration of these drugs especially when mixed with alcohol ('spiked drinks') produce disinhibition and lasting anterograde amnesia for the events that occur under the influence of the drug, making the victim an unreliable witness. Because symptoms caused by these agents mimic those of alcohol, not all victims are screened for their presence [71, 72].

Flunitrazepam is a potent benzodiazepine. When dissolved in a drink, it is odorless and tasteless, and produces symptoms similar to alcohol intoxication and should be suspected in any sexual assault involving a person who appears intoxicated or has amnesia [73].

GHB ('liquid ecstasy') is a metabolite of the inhibitory neurotransmitter gamma-aminobutyric acid, acting as a central nervous system depressant. GHB is colorless and odorless but may have a distinct salty taste. In small doses, it lowers inhibition and instills feelings of euphoria. In higher doses, it produces drowsiness, amnesia, confusion and hallucinations. These symptoms can be accompanied by nausea and vomiting [73].

Ketamine hydrochloride is a rapid-acting nonopioid, lipid soluble anesthetic with a short elimination half-life. It produces a state of 'dissociative anesthesia', probably from action on N-methyl-D-aspartate receptors. The psychotropic effects of ketamine range from dissociation and depersonalization to psychotic experiences and include a sensation of feeling light, body distortion, absence of the sense of time, novel experiences of cosmic oneness and out of body experiences [74]. If mixed in alcoholic drinks, a synergistic effect is obtained.

Despite of all the media coverage, the real use of the above substances appears to be low. Of 2003 urine samples collected by rape treatment centers in the US, in cases of suspicion of drug-facilitated rape, GHB was detected only in 3% of the samples and flunitrazepam in less than 1%. Nevertheless, alcohol was detected in 69% of the samples, marijuana in 18% and cocaine in 5% [75]. In a similar study, Indmarch and Brinkman [70] in the UK tested 1,033 samples. Nearly 20 different substances were detected among the 611 specimens that tested positive – 37% were positive for alcohol, 18.5% were positive for cannabinoids, GHB was detected in 4.4% of samples, and only 0.6% showed evidence of flunitrazepam.

This evidence does not point to the widespread use of these substances as 'date rape drugs'. If we broaden the concept of 'rape drug' to any substance that is administered to lower sexual inhibition and enhance the possibility of unwanted sexual intercourse, the principal suspect for a drug-facilitated rape would be alcohol [73].

Guidelines and procedures should be established to ensure that forensic samples are collected following the allegations of possible drug-mediated sexual assault [76].

Drugs and Risky Behavior

Particularly after the AIDS epidemic, health authorities became aware of the necessity of implementing measures to control the spread of STDs. In this context, researchers soon began to investigate the impairments in the practice of safer sex and, among many other hypotheses, they conjectured about the use of safe sex practices among people who were using mind-altering substances.

Thus, a considerable amount of research on the relationship of sexuality and drugs deals with the spread of HIV- and hepatitis-associated drug abuse and community efforts to prevent these infections [77].

Could the use of these substances cloud the good judgment about a possible sexual situation in which the drug user is involved? Would people under drugs be less able to use safety measures regarding STDs? Or perhaps drug users are at risk not because of their drug use, but because of the characteristics of their personality?

First of all, it must be established that drug users do have a sex life. Sometimes, clinicians in drug therapy settings know that chronic use of drugs severely impairs sexuality and consequently they tend to disregard the sex life of their clients. Goldberg et al. [78] stated that drug injectors with serious opiate and tranquilizer dependency are at least as sexually active as the general population.

Our research [37] shows that, at least for opioid-addicted men, there is a decrease in sexual activity, but the fact is that the majority of drug users, including drug injectors, are sexuality active with their partners or, in significant minority (mostly women) involved in prostitution [79].

Although some addicts may be reducing their HIV risk, abandoning the sharing of injecting equipment or the IV use altogether, they may maintain some risky sexual behavior [80]. The levels of condom use, even for drug injectors, are low and inconsistent for both men and women [37, 79, 81].

The risk of HIV transmission among nonintravenous drug users is likely to be related to sexual transmission of HIV, particularly due to the prevalence of high-risk sexual behavior and STDs in this population [82].

Addicted women are more likely to have a sex partner who is a drug user and also to be living with a drug user [83]. The same is not true for addicted men who, in many instances, have a healthy female for a sex companion or are living with a healthy female [84]. The sexual risks involved vary, of course, with these different situations.

Healthy female partners of male drug users in stable relationships, although theoretically knowing the risks involved in using drugs may feel as though that risk would not apply to their partnership and act accordingly with a very low use of safety measures against STDs [84].

In this way, drug users can be at risk for STDs or putting at risk their sex partners as there are relatively high levels of sexual mixing between drug injectors and noninjectors [79] and between drug users and nonusers [84].

Prostitution can be a source of income for drug addicts [79]. In a recent study, we found [9] a significant number of female drug addicts engaging in prostitution activities, and the age at which these activities began correlated with the age at which they began the daily use of drugs.

In this money for sex exchange, it seems that STD prevention is uncommon. High levels of unprotected anal intercourse are found among prostitutes and drug users [85].

As prostitution activities in this population are mostly drug driven, treatment of drug dependence can have a positive effect on that behavior. Meandzija et al. [86] showed that the intravenous drug users they studied engaged in high-risk sexual behaviors, but methadone maintenance reduced sex for drugs or money exchange.

In fact, treatment may be crucial for reducing sexual risk in drug addicts, but it may be necessary to increase or find new strategies for risk prevention, as some studies show that there is no association between treatment and safer sexual practices [87]. A longer treatment career may be effective as Longshore and Hsieh [88] demonstrated that users with more lifetime treatment exposure had lower scores for risky sex. This is consistent with the hypothesis that successive episodes of treatment may have long-term cumulative effects on drug users' HIV risk behavior.

Until now, we have been discussing problems related to drug dependence, but we must now consider the influence of acute drug use and its possible influence on decision making regarding risky sex situations.

It would be reasonable to assume that the use of a mind-altering substance prior to sexual activity may result in impaired decision making about the whole situation, including prevention of STDs.

Research has shown that substance use (including alcohol, marijuana, methamphetamines and others) prior to or during sex, is a significant predictor of high-risk sexual behavior, regardless of sex, age, ethnicity or sexual orientation [5, 64, 89].

Nevertheless, some studies do not support the assumption of a casual relationship between substance abuse and risky sex even in high-risk samples [90]. In Scotland, Leigh and Miller [91] in a sample of more than 1,300 respondents from urban areas, examined alcohol or drug use in conjunction with sexual activity and the use of condoms and other contraceptives and concluded that people combining sex with alcohol or drugs are not necessarily more likely to engage in riskier sex.

Miller et al. [92] investigated risk taking related to sex and drug use to find that this behavior was neither entirely general nor entirely specific with distinct types of risk taking being distinguished.

Results from the study by Schafer et al. [93], support an association between drug use (other than alcohol) and decreased likelihood of condom use with a new sexual partner. Individuals who used drugs and did not use condoms scored significantly higher on a scale assessing impulsivity, risk taking and sensation seeking.

An explanation for the resistance or inability to change sexual risky behaviors among drug users has been advanced by Singer [94]. This author proposes that sexual risk behavior may be understood and explained in the context of clients' perception of themselves and their relationships, as a result of past traumatic events and current lifestyle.

There is sufficient evidence for considering that using drugs before or during sexual intercourse can, in certain circumstances, put the parts involved at risk of unwanted pregnancy or STDs. Prevention programs directed at occasional users of recreational drugs and risk prevention for drug addicts and their sex partners are thus a matter of health priority.

Drugs Used as Sexual Aids

Drugs of abuse can sometimes be used as sexual aids. A study by Maroli et al. [6], found that 20% of the interviewed sample made use of alcohol, cannabis, cocaine and other drugs of abuse specifically with sexual purposes.

In a general population study in the US, with ages ranging from 18 to 39 years, Foxman et al. [95] found that 13% had used some drug to enhance sexual experience. The most commonly used drugs were alcohol (83.7%), marijuana (34.7%), ecstasy or 'sextasy' (8.2%) and sildenafil (7.5%).

In some cases, drugs may be used to increase sexual performance in the absence of a real sexual problem, but in other cases drug use can be seen as a self-medication for a previous and not diagnosed sexual dysfunction.

This has been called *La Pera hypothesis*, according to which, a very large percentage of young people begin the use of drugs due to sexual problems. To validate this hypothesis, La Pera et al. [96] conducted a research in rehabilitation centers for drug addicts and found out that 50% of the entire sample used psychotropic drugs to improve their sexual performance. 34% stated that their sexual disorder has influenced their decision to start taking drugs (among these 13.3% considered it had been a decisive factor).

Confirming this hypothesis, the study by Palha and Esteves [50], completed in 2007, established a relation between depression and sexual complaints in heroin addicts. Some individuals in this sample presented important anxiety and phobic symptoms; the severity of these positively correlated with the age at first sexual intercourse and number of sexual partners through life.

Among the use of drugs during sex with the intent to increase performance or pleasure we could include alcohol, amphetamines, cocaine and ecstasy, whose effects were described above. Other substances are sometimes used that are of interest for the clinician.

Lignocaine, although not in itself a drug of abuse, is sometimes used in a spray form for delaying ejaculation. As it is an anesthetic, it will give a dull sensation not only in the subject's penis, but also in the areas of the partner receiving it [3].

Vasodilators (butyl nitrate, glyceryl trinitrate, amyl nitrate and isosorbide dinitrate) are known as 'poppers' and presented in small bottles or ampoules. Their vapors liberate nitrous oxide. The users describe a sensation of 'rush', followed by euphoria, with intensification of positive emotions. As nitrous oxide is a muscle relaxant, it is used sometimes to facilitate anal intercourse. It is suspected, but without a solid evidence, that these drugs can depress the immune system [3].

Cocaine applied on the penis glands or on the clitoris acts as a local anesthetic delaying orgasm. Placed in the anus its anesthetic effect can facilitate anal coitus with the danger, however, of preventing pain in dangerous insertions [3].

Sextasy is the common name for a drug combination of ecstasy and sildenafil which is a phosphodiesterase-5 inhibitor used for the pharmacological treatment of erectile dysfunction. Sildenafil is sometimes also used in conjunction with other street drugs like cocaine, cannabis or 'poppers' [97, 98]. The users of this dangerous combination report enhanced sexual desire and love making and feelings of 'warmth'. About a half report negative effects: headaches, genital soreness and intoxication. Cases of priapism have also been reported [97].

Bearing in mind the vasoactive properties of the drugs involved (sildenafil and 'poppers' in particular), there is a serious risk of a possible cardiovascular accident (drop of blood pressure, myocardial infarction or stroke) [97].

Management

Sex life is seldom questioned in clinical settings. Therefore, the first task would be making health professionals more aware of the importance of assessing the sex life of their patients. This is more so in addiction medicine, where failing to understand the sexual difficulties of dependents may induce relapses or losing therapeutic opportunities.

Singer et al. [99] studied the impact of tailored training courses on sexual counseling addressed to drug workers. Attitudinal changes took place. Training appeared to have increased the staff's awareness of the importance of sexual counseling and reduced the perceived difficulty of discussing certain specific sexual issues.

The diagnoses of psychotropic drug-induced sexual function disorders are easy to establish if the psychiatrist is sensitive to the existence of these adverse effects. This mostly involves careful history taking, although several questionnaires have been developed for reliable and valid quantification of sexual functioning. Diagnosis is usually established if the sexual function disorders develop when the patient is using a psychotropic drug and then disappear when the offending drug is discontinued [100].

Checcucci [8] described an intervention method to promote a sound and nondestructive sexuality. This method is proposed for therapeutic communities, where the patients are abstinent and in a specific environment providing an opportunity to establish numerous human relations and experiment new lifestyles and roles. Here, the theme of sexuality is included in a wider context including affectivity, family life and personality traits of the users, re-elaborating the whole history, enabling them to use it in a healthier way in the future, and preventing it from becoming a destructive tool. The work is carried out in small groups and comprises three levels of intervention: *Providing information* in most aspects of sexuality and the links between sexuality and drugs; *process of liberation*, understanding, sharing and accepting one's past, identifying personal problems and discussing how to cope with them, and *process of elaboration and reorientation* – clarifying the material emerged and using it to adopt new lifestyles.

We propose that professional addiction training should have some teaching sessions on clinical sexology and conversely clinical sexology training should have some addiction insights. We also think that it is useful to have at least one trained clinical sexologist in the addiction unit.

References

1 Sandroni P: Aphrodisiacs past and present: s historical review. Clin Auton Res 2000;11:303–307.
2 Nordenberg T: The facts about aphrodisiacs. FDA Consum 1996;30:10–15.
3 Headon C, Huish M: Sex aids; in Tomlinson J (ed): ABC of Sexual Health. London, BMJ Books, 1999.
4 Smith S: Drugs that cause sexual dysfunction. Psychiatry 2007;6:111–114.
5 Staton M, Leukefeld C, Logan TK, Zimmerman R, Lynam D, Milich R, Martin C, McClanahan K, Clayton R: Risky sex behavior and substance use among young adults. Ment Soc Work 1999;24:147–154.
6 Maroli A, Forza G, Schifano F: Indagine conoscitiva su uso di sostanze psicoattive e sessualità. Boll Farmacodip Alcolis 2000;23:32–40.
7 Saso L: Effetti delle sostanze d'abuso sulla risposta sessuale. Ann Ist Super Sanità 2002;38:289–294.
8 Checcucci G: Sexuality and drug addiction: A tailored intervention during a rehabilitation program in a therapeutic community. Ital J Drug Addict Alcohol 2002;24:1–2.
9 Esteves MF: Depressão e toxicodependência- influência da patologia depressiva na evolução da síndrome de dependência dos opiáceos. Porto, MEDISA, Edições e Divulgações Científicas Ldª, 2005.
10 Rosenbaum M: When drugs come into the picture, love flies out the window: Women addicts' love relationships. Int J Addict 1981;16:1197–1206.
11 McKay A: Sexuality and substance use: The impact of tobacco, alcohol and selected recreational drugs on sexual function. Can J Hum Sex 2005;14:47–56.
12 Gordon GG, Southren AL, Vittek J, Lieber CS: The effect of alcohol ingestion on hepatic aromatase activity and plasma steroid hormones in the rat. Metabolism 1979;28:20–24.
13 Lieber CS: Hepatic and metabolic effects of ethanol: Pathogenesis and prevention. Ann Med 1994;26: 325–330.
14 Gavaler JS, Rosenblum ER, Deal SR, Bowie BT: The phytoestrogen congeners of alcohol beverages: Current status. Proc Soc Exp Biol Med 1995;208: 98–102.
15 Calabrese G: Nonalcoholic compounds of wine: the phytoestrogen resveratrol and moderate red wine consumption during menopause. Drugs Exp Clin Res 1999;25:111–114.
16 Nordmann R, Ribiere C, Rouach H: Ethanol-induced lipid peroxidation and oxidative stress in extrahepatic tissues. Alcohol Alcohol 1990;25:231–237.
17 Rivier C, Rivest S, Vale W: Alcohol-induced inhibition of LH secretion in intact and gonadectomized male and femal rats: Possible mechanisms. Alcohol Clin Exp Res 1992;16:935–941.
18 Silva SM, Madeira MD, Ruela C, Paula-Barbosa MM: Prolonged alcohol intake leads to irreversible loss of vasopressin and oxytocin neurons in the paraventricular nucleus of the hypothalamus. Brain Res 2002;925:76–88.
19 Carmichael MS, Humbert R, Dixen J, Palmisano G, Greenleaf W, Davidson JM: Plasma oxytocin increases in the human sexual response. J Clin Endocrinol Metab 1987;64:27–31.
20 Blaicher W, Gruber D, Bieglmayer C, Blaicher AM, Knogler W, Huber JC: The role of oxytocin in relation to female sexual arousal. Gynecol Obstet Invest 1999;47:125–126.
21 Derby CA, Mohr BA, Goldstein I, Felman HA, Johanes CB, McKinlay JB: Modifiable risk factors and erectile dysfunction; can lifestyle changes modify risk? Urology 2000;56:302–306.

22 Feldman HA, Johannes CB, Derby CA, Kleinman KP, Mohr BA, Araujo AB, McKinley JB: Erectile dysfunction and coronary risk factors: prospective results from the Massachusettes Male Aging Study. Prev Med 2000;30:328–338.
23 Dorey G: Is smoking a cause of erectile dysfunction? A literature review. Br J Nurs 2001;10:455–465.
24 Gades NM, Nehra A, Jacobson DJ, McGree ME, Girman CJ, Rhodes T, Roberts RO, Lieber MM, Jacobsen SJ: Association between smoking and erectile dysfunction: A population-based study. Am J Epidemiol 2005;161:346–351.
25 Natali A, Mondaini N, Lombardi G, Del Popolo, Rizzo M: Heavy smoking is an important risk factor for erectile dysfunction in young men. Int J Impot Res 2004;17:227–330.
26 Sullivan ME, Keoghane SR, Miller MAW: Vascular risk factors and erectile dycfunction. Br J Urol 2001;87:838–845.
27 Wolf R, Shulman A: Erectile dysfunction and fertility related to cigarette smoking. J Eur Acad Dermatol Venereol 1996;6:209–216.
28 Pourmand G, Alidaee MR, Rasuli S, Maleki A, Mehrsai A: Do cigarette smokers with erectile dysfunction benefit from stopping?: A prospective study. BJU Int 2004;94:1310–1313.
29 Iversen LL: The science of marijuana. New York: Oxford University Press, 2000.
30 Halikas J, Weller R, Morse C: Effects of regular marijuana use on sexual performance. J Psychoactive Drugs 1982;14:59–70.
31 Rosen RC: Alcohol and drug effects on sexual response: human experimental and clinical studies. Annu Rev Sex Res 1991;2:119–179.
32 Smith DE, Moser C, Wesson DR, Apter M, Buxton ME, Davison JV, Orgel M, Buffum JA: A clinical guide to the diagnoses and treatment of heroin-related sexual dysfunction. J Psychoactive Drugs 1982;14:91–99.
33 King VL, Brooner RK, Bigelow GE, Schmidt CW, Felch LJ, Gazaway PM: Condom use rates for specific sexual behaviors among opioid abusers entering treatment. Drug Alcohol Depend 1994;35:231–238.
34 Cushman P: Sexual behavior in heroin addiction and methadone maintenance. NY State J Med 1972;72:1261–1265.
35 Mintz J, O'Hare K, O'Brien CP, Goldschmidt CW: Sexual problems of heroin addicts. Arch Gen Psychiatry 1974;137:909–915.
36 Masters WM, Johnson VE, Kolodny RC: Masters and Johnson on Sex and Human Loving. Boston, Little Brown, 1986.
37 Palha AP, Esteves MF: A study of the sexuality of opiate addicts. J Sex Marital Ther 2002;28:427–437.
38 Wang C, Chan V, Yeung RT: The effect of heroin addiction on pituitary-testicular function. Clin Endocrinol (Oxf) 1978;9:455–461.
39 Lafisca S, Bolelli G, Franceschetti F, Danieli A, Tagliaro F, Magiro M, Flamigni C: Free and bound testosterone in male heroin addicts. Arch Toxicol Suppl 1985;8:394–397.
40 Malik SA, Khan C, Jabbar A, Iqbal A: Heroin addiction and sex hormones in males. J Pak Med Assoc 1992;42:210–212.
41 Roberts L, Finch PM, Pullan P, Bhagat C, Price LM: Sex hormone suppression by intrathecal opioids: A prospective study. Clin J Pain 2002;18:144–148.
42 Mendelson JH, Meyer RE, Ellingboe J, Mirin SM, McDougle M: Effects of heroin and methadone on plasma cortisol and testosterone. J Pharmacol Exp Ther 1975;195:296–302.
43 Chessick RD: The 'pharmacogenic orgasm' in the drug addict. Arch Gen Psychiatry 1960;3:545–556.
44 Seecof R, Tennant FS: Subjective perceptions to the intravenous 'rush' of heroin and cocaine in opioid addicts. Am J Drug Alcohol Abuse 1986;12:79–87.
45 Bozarth MA: Pleasure systems in the brain; in Warburton DM (ed): Pleasure: The politics and the reality. New York, John Wiley & Sons, 1994, pp 5–14+refs.
46 Redmond DE Jr, Kosten TR, Reiser, MF: Spontaneous ejaculation associated with anxiety: psychopathological considerations. Am J Psychiatry 1983; 140:1163–1166.
47 Cushman P, Dole VP: Detoxification of rehabilitated methadone-maintenance patients. J Am Med Assoc 1973;226:747–752.
48 VanAhlen H, Piechota HJ, Kias J, Brennemann W, Klingmuller D: Opiate antagonists in erectile dysfunction: a possible new treatment option? Results from a pilot study with naltrexone. Eur Urol 1995;28:246–250.
49 Sathe RS, Komisaruk BR, Ladas AK, Godbole SV: Naltrexone-induced augmentation of sexual response in men. Arch Med Res 2001;32:221–226.
50 Palha AP, Esteves MF: Co-morbilidade psiquiátrica e função sexual em dependentes de opiáceos. Arquivos de Psiquiatria 2008; in press.
51 Peugh MA, Belenko S: Alcohol, drugs, and sexual function: a review. J Psychoactive Drugs 2001;33: 223–232.
52 MacDonald PT, Waldorf D, Reinarman C, Murphy S: Heavy cocaine use and sexual behavior. J Drug Issues 1988;18:437–455.
53 Wetherby NL, Shultz JM, Chitwood DD, McCoy HV, McCoy CV, Ludwig DD, Edlin BR: Crack cocaine use and sexual activity in Miami, Florida. J Psychoactive Drugs 1992;24:373–380.

54 Henderson DJ, Boyd CJ, Whitmarsh J: Women and illicit drugs: sexuality and crack cocaine. Health Care Women Int 1995;16:113–124.

55 Mireku-Boateng DJ, Tasie B: Priapism associated with intracavernosal injection of cocaine. Urol Int 2001;67:109–110.

56 Maxwell JC: Emerging research on methamphetamine. Curr Opin Psychiatry 2005;18:235–242.

57 Fiorino DF, Phillips AG: Facilitation of sexual behavior in male rats following d-amphetamine-induced behavioral sensitization. Psychopharmacol 1999;142:200–208.

58 Gossop MR, Stern R, Connel PH: Drug dependence and sexual dysfunction: a comparison of intravenous users of narcotics and oral users of amphetamines. Br J Psychiatry 1974;124:431–434.

59 Hafen BQ, Soulier D: Amphetamines. Facts, figures and information. Hazelden PES, 1990.

60 Semple SJ, Patterson TL, Grant I: The context of sexual risk behavior among heterosexual methamphetamine users. Addict Behav 2004;29:807–810.

61 Kurtz SP: Post-circuit blues: Motivations and consequences of crystal meth use among gay men in Miami. AIDS Behav 2005;9:63–72.

62 Frosch D, Shoptaw S, Huber A, Rawson RA, Ling W: Sexual HIV risk among gay and bisexual male methamphetamine abusers. J Subst Abuse Treat 1996;13:483–486.

63 Hirshfield S, Remien RH, Walavalker I, Chiasson MA: Crystal methamphetamine use predicts incident STD infection among men who have sex with men recruited online: A nested case-control study. J Med Internet Res 2004;6:e41.

64 Molitor F, Truax SR, Ruiz JD, Sun R: Association of methanphetamine use during sex with risky sexual behaviors and HIV infection among non-injection drug users. West J Med 1998;168:93–97.

65 Steele TD, McCann UD, Ricaurte GA: 3,4 – methylenedioxymethamphetamine (MDMA, 'Ecstasy'): pharmacology and toxicology in animals and humans. Addiction 1994;89:539–551.

66 Schiavi RC, Segraves RT: The biology of sexual function. Psychiatr Clin North Am 1995;18:7–23.

67 Zemishlany Z, Aizenberg D, Weizman A: Subjective effects of MDMA ('Ecstasy') on human sexual function. Eur Psychiatry 2001;16:127–130.

68 Buffum J, Moser C: MDMA and human sexual function. J Psychoactive Drugs 1986;18:355–359.

69 Dublin N, Razack AH: Priapism: ecstasy related? Urology 2000;56:1057.

70 Indmarch I, Brinkman R: Trends in the use of alcohol and other drugs in cases of sexual assault. Human Psychopharmacology: Clin Experiment 1999; 14:225–231.

71 Smith KM: Drugs used in acquaintance rape. J Am Pharm Assoc (Wash) 1999;39:442–443.

72 Schwartz RH, Milteer R, LeBeau MA: Drug-facilitated sexual assault ('date rape'). South Med J 2000;94:655–656.

73 Weir E: Drug-facilitated date rape. J de l'Assoc Méd Can 2001;165:80.

74 Pal HR, Berry N, Kumar R, Ray R: Ketamine dependence. Anaesth Intensive Care 2002;30:382–384.

75 Slaughter L: Involvement of drugs in sexual assault. J Reprod Med 2000;45:425–430.

76 Indmarch I, ElSohly J, Gambles J, Salamone S: Forensic urinalysis of drug use in cases of alleged sexual assault. J Clin Forensic Med 2001;8:197–205.

77 Battjes RJ, Leukefeld CG, Amsel Z: Community prevention efforts to reduce the spread of AIDS associated with intravenous drug abuse; in Battjes RJ, Leukefeld CG, Amsel Z: AIDS and Intravenous Drug Use: Future Directions for Community-Based Prevention Research. Rockville, NIDA Research Monograph, 1990, pp 288–298.

78 Goldberg D, Frischer M, Green ST: Sex surveys and drug users. Nature 1993;361:504–505.

79 Rhodes T, Stimson GV, Quirk, A: Sex, drugs, intervention and research: from the individual to the social. Subst Use Misuse 1996;31:375–407.

80 Donoghoe MC: Sex, HIV and the injecting drug user. Br J Addict 1992;87:405–416.

81 Schilling RF, el Bassel N, Schinke SP, Nichols S, Botvin GJ, Orlandi MA: Sexual behavior, attitudes toward safer sex, and gender among a cohort of 244 recovering IV drug users. Int J Addict 1991;26: 859–877.

82 Lehman JS, Allen DM, Green TA, Onorato IM: HIV infection among non-injecting drug users entering drug treatment, United States, 1989–1992. AIDS 1994;8:1465–1469.

83 Gossop M, Griffiths P, Strang J: Sex differences in patterns of drug taking behavior. Br J Psychiatry 1994;164:101–104.

84 Brito M: Relações perigosas. As companheiras de dependentes de opiáceos: Contribuição para o seu estudo. Master of Sciences Dissertation. Faculty of Psychology, University of Oporto, 1997.

85 Powis B, Griffiths P, Gossop M, Strang J: Heterosexual anal intercourse, health risks and drug use: A review with special attention to drug users. Drug Alcohol Rev 1995;14:223–229.

86 Meandzija B, O'Connor PG, Fitzgerald B, Rounsaville BJ, Kosten TR: HIV infection and cocaine use in methadone maintained and untreated intravenous drug users. Drug Alcohol Depend 1994;36: 109–113.

87 Darke S, Hall W, Carless J: Drug use, injecting practices and sexual behavior of opioid users in Sydney, Australia. Br J Addict 1990;85:1603–1609.
88 Longshore D, Hsieh S: Drug abuse treatment and risky sex: evidence for a cumulative treatment effect? Am J Drug Alcohol Abuse 1998;24:439–451.
89 Mulry G, Kalichman SC, Kelly JA: Substance use and unsafe sex among gay men: Global versus situational use of substances. J Sex Educ Ther 1994;20: 175–184.
90 Baker SA, Morrison DM, Gillmore MR, Schock, MD: Sexual behaviors, substance use, and condom use in a sexually transmitted disease clinic sample. J Sex Res 1995;32:37–44.
91 Leigh B, Miller P: The relationship of substance use with sex to the use of condoms among young adults in two urban areas of Scotland. AIDS Educ Prev 1995;7:278–284.
92 Miller P, Plant M, Plant M, Duffy J: Alcohol, tobacco, illicit drugs and sex: An analysis of risky behaviors among young adults. Int J Addict 1995;30: 239–258.
93 Schafer J, Blanchard L, Fals SW: Drug use and risky sexual behavior. Psychol Addict Behav 1994; 8:3–7.
94 Singer N: Understanding sexual risk behavior from drug user's accounts of their life experiences. Qual Health Res 1995;5:237–249.
95 Foxman B, Aral SO, Holmes KK: Common use in the general population of sexual enrichment aids and drugs to enhance sexual experience. Sex Transm Dis 2006;33:156–162.
96 La Pera G, Carderi A, Mariantantoni Z, Lentini M, Taggi F: The role of sexualdysfunctions in inducing the use of drug in young males. Arch Ital Urol Androl 2006;78:101–106.
97 Aldridge J, Measham F: Sildenafil (Viagra) is used as a recreational drug in England. Br Med J 1999; 318:669.
98 Breslau K: The 'sextasy' craze. Clubland's dangerous aprty mix: Viagra and extasy. Newsweek 2007; Oct 29.
99 Singer N, Phillips K, White D, Mulleady G, Whitehead B: Evaluation of a training course on sexual counseling in a drug work setting. AIDS Care 1994; 6:221–235.
100 Clayton DO, Shen WW: Psychotropic drug-induced sexual function disorders: Diagnoses, incidence and management. Drug Saf 1998;19:299–312.

A. Pacheco-Palha, MD, PhD
Rua do Carvalho, 109-4EA
PT–4150-192 Porto (Portugal)
Tel. +351 226 185 153, Fax +351 225 512 334, E-Mail apalha@sapo.pt

Balon R (ed): Sexual Dysfunction. The Brain-Body Connection.
Adv Psychosom Med. Basel, Karger, 2008, vol 29, pp 150–168

Contribution of Imaging to Our Understanding of Sexual Function and Dysfunction

Terri L. Woodard · Michael P. Diamond

Division of Reproductive Endocrinology and Infertility, Department of Obstetrics and Gynecology, Wayne State University School of Medicine, Detroit, Mich., USA

Abstract

The physiology of sexual function and dysfunction is complex and involves biologic, psychological, emotional and social factors in both men and women. As a result, multiple investigative tools are needed to achieve a thorough and comprehensive understanding of these processes. Recently, there have been many advances in the field of medical imaging; many of these imaging techniques have been applied to the study of sexual function and have allowed us to obtain an additional perspective of sexual processes in the research setting. The purpose of this chapter is to review and discuss these techniques with an emphasis on how they contribute to our understanding of sexual function and dysfunction.

Sexual function (and dysfunction), though of utmost importance to the process of reproduction and general quality of life, has been difficult for us to completely understand. While there has always been an interest in the topic of sex, most major advances in the field of sexology have been recent. Certainly, we have achieved an improved understanding of male sexual physiology – particularly about the physiology and treatment of male erectile dysfunction (ED) using sildenafil. However, with regard to female sexual physiology, we have a much poorer understanding, though notable attempts are being made to elucidate the involved mechanisms.

One of the major problems with understanding sexual function is that it is a complex entity that involves many processes, including biological, psychological, emotional and social factors. Hence, it is doubtful that the study of one particular process can tell us everything we need to know about sexual functioning; accordingly, it is just as unlikely that any single investigative tool can provide a comprehensive explanation. Given the multidimensional nature of sexual function, multiple, diverse instruments need to be utilized to maximize our understanding. These instruments include but are not limited to psychophysiologic modalities such as the vaginal photoplethysmograph (a small, tampon-shaped device which is inserted into the vagina and measures vaginal blood volume and vaginal pulse amplitude in response to an erotic stimulus) and RigiScan (an instrument that measures penile tumescence and rigidity), as well as validated questionnaires designed to assess sexual function and dysfunction.

There have been considerable advances in medical imaging over the past few decades, including the development of laser Doppler perfusion imaging (LDPI) and functional magnetic resonance imaging (fMRI). Researchers have begun applying these techniques to the study of sexual function and dysfunction. Though such imaging studies are not widely used in the clinical arena and are mainly employed in the research setting, they are giving us new insight about sexual processes. In the field of sex research, imaging studies have been used to describe the anatomy of sexual intercourse, study the anatomy of genital structures over the course of the sexual response cycle and in response to various treatments and interventions, and to assess the brain structures that are involved in sexual desire, arousal and orgasm. In this chapter, we will review and discuss these various techniques and what they have and may potentially contribute to our understanding of male and female sexual function. The use of imaging in sex research is a challenging, yet exciting and promising endeavor that may potentially enable us to improve our ability to assist and treat individuals with sexual dysfunction.

Imaging of Intercourse

Over 500 years ago, Leonardo da Vinci created a piece entitled, *The Copulation*, which was his rendition of what intercourse looks like anatomically. In the male, he constructed a tract from the spinal cord to the penis, which apparently carried semen. Notably, the penis is drawn as a straight organ. In the female, he depicts a tract running from the breast to the vagina. Though obviously anatomically incorrect, his rendition was likely influenced by the social thoughts of his time [1]. However, it was Robert Dickinson, commonly regarded as one of the first great American sexologists, who first utilized a scientific approach to describe coital anatomy. He used a glass tube shaped like an erect penis to simulate coitus in sexually aroused women; using this model, he drew anatomical pictures of coitus and postulated that the penis preferentially contacts the posterior fornix of the vagina [2]. In the 1960s, Masters and Johnson used artificial penises to delineate coital anatomy using gynecologic speculums and bimanual examination. Their most notable findings were the phenomenon of 'vaginal tenting' (the back and upwards displacement of the anterior vagina during intercourse) and a reported increase in uterine volume by 50–100% [3].

It has been and continues to be a challenge to assess the anatomical and physiologic changes that occur during coitus. While there are some studies that used MRI to assess the distribution of contraceptive gels during intercourse [4], relatively few devoted strictly to coital anatomy exist. Social, ethical and logistical barriers make the execution of such studies quite difficult. However, the few studies that exist were devised to test the hypotheses of the past and give us a better glimpse into the anatomic changes that occur during coitus.

Ultrasound

There have been very few studies using ultrasound to assess coital anatomy and physiology. In 1992, Riley et al. [5] used ultrasound to assess an intravaginal barrier contraceptive during human coitus in 10 couples. In 9 out of 10 couples, they noted an indentation and stretching of the anterior wall of the vagina and no direct impact on the posterior wall in any coital position. In 2 out of 9 couples engaged in a rear-entry position, there was cervical impact. However, this study was limited by extremely poor-quality images. Furthermore, the subjects were required to self-scan, which may have interfered with coital positioning and achievement of optimal sexual performance.

Deng et al. [6] reported their experience using real-time volumetric ultrasound with minimal compression to evaluate the functional anatomy of the penis during erection and simulated coitus in a water bath. They recruited 5 men to participate in the study; after the first subject was unable to achieve an adequate erection, the investigators devised a gel vagina, placed in the water bath to help achieve adequate stimulation for erection. Using this new device, the subsequent subjects were able to complete the study. The investigators were able to visualize sonographic changes in penile anatomic structures, including a decreased echogenic intensity in the corpus cavernosum from baseline to the erect state. They postulated that these were a result of microvascular changes within the penis.

Ultrasound could potentially be a useful adjunct to the study of coital physiology because it allows coitus to be studied in 'real-time', it is relatively noninvasive and inexpensive. However it is limited by poor resolution and variability in measurements due to operator-dependent characteristics. While the volumetric ultrasound with minimal compression appears to circumvent some of these limitations and yields potentially meaningful data in men, it is not readily adapted for use in women.

Magnetic Resonance Imaging

In 1999, Schultz et al. [7] set out to determine the feasibility of using MRI to study coitus. They performed a descriptive study of 13 experiments on 8 couples and 3 women. To allow both partners to fit in the MRI machine, they removed the table to achieve a tube diameter of 50 cm. Using a Siemens 1.5-tesla MRI machine, images were taken of the female pelvis at baseline, of the couple in the missionary position, and of the women alone during and after masturbation to orgasm. Key findings were that the penis is shaped like a boomerang and the uterus does not increase in volume, contrary to the depiction of the penis by da Vinci or the findings of Masters and

Johnson. A few years later, Faix also used MRI, which revealed that in the missionary position, there was preferential contact of the penis with the anterior vaginal wall and anterior fornix [8]. In a subsequent study, MRI was used to study anatomical differences during coitus between two different positions in the same couple [9]. They found that in the missionary position, the penis reached the anterior fornix with preferential contact of the anterior vaginal wall. The posterior bladder was pushed forward and the uterus was pushed upward and backward. During the rear-entry position, the penis reached the posterior fornix with preferential contact of the posterior vaginal wall, with the bladder and uterus pushed forward. They suggested that female genital stimulation may have a strong positional influence that is dependent on the coital position of the vaginal and uterine axis.

MRI is advantageous because it permits observation of the anatomy of coitus with better resolution and detail than ultrasonography, though in the above studies the resolution was not high enough to adequately see other structures that may play a role in sexual function, such as the urethra and the erectile tissue of the vestibular bulbs. In addition, MRI is expensive, time-consuming and scanner availability is often limited. Furthermore, sexual performance may be inhibited in the scanner environment; in the Schultz study [7], the use of sildenafil was required on several occasions to achieve adequate erection in the males; additionally, females reported their orgasms as being more 'superficial' than those experienced in their normal environment. Finally, the limited number of subjects involved in these studies make it difficult to apply these findings to the general population. While the findings from the MRI studies are intriguing and they describe coital anatomy in an objective way, they raise more questions than they answer. More studies will need to be done before its clinical application is a relevant and practical possibility.

Anatomical Imaging

Imaging has been used to provide anatomical information about specific genital structures with regard to sexual function. The use of imaging in men has centered mainly on ED; with better therapies for ED available, the use of imaging in the routine diagnostic workup of ED has decreased substantially. However, ultrasound and MRI are being used. In more complex cases where surgery may be an option, cavernosography and pudendal arteriograms may be indicated. Given their limited use and invasiveness, these will not be discussed here. Because of the lack of understanding of female sexual function as well as the difficulty of diagnosis and treatment of female sexual dysfunction disorders, there are a greater number of imaging modalities that have been explored with hopes of elucidating these mechanisms, including ultrasonography, MRI, LDPI and thermography. Pudendal arteriograms have also been used for diagnostic purposes in a limited number of cases [10], but will not be discussed in this review.

Ultrasound

Doppler ultrasonography uses standard ultrasound methods to produce a picture of blood vessels and surrounding organs. A computer converts the Doppler sounds into a graph that provides information about the speed and direction of blood flow through the blood vessel being evaluated. This modality was first used to evaluate female genital hemodynamics by Lavoisier et al. [11] in 1995 to measure clitoral blood flow. Ten healthy women were recruited in this study. A clitoral artery was found and the signal was allowed to stabilize. Without moving the ultrasound probe, a pressure probe inflated to 100 mg Hg was inserted into the lower 1/3 vagina and taken out after 20–30 s. This was repeated several times and the pressure was increased in the pressure probe. Only 2 out of the 8 women reported any degree of subjective sexual arousal. They showed that clitoral blood flow increased in response to vaginal pressure stimulation. Using ultrasound, investigators have also shown that in normal women, clitoral blood flow increases significantly after topical administration of 0.2% alprostadil gel [12]. Subsequently, another study showed that there is a difference in clitoral peak systolic and end diastolic velocity after topical administration of alprostadil between women with sexual dysfunction versus healthy controls, implying a potential diagnostic role of topical vasoactive agents in ultrasound evaluation of women with sexual dysfunction [13].

Berman et al. [14] used Duplex Doppler ultrasound to measure clitoral, labial, urethral and vaginal arterial peak systolic velocity and end diastolic velocity of 48 women presenting with sexual complaints. These measurements were taken at baseline and following stimulation with a 15-min erotic video and vibrator. It was observed that sexual stimulation resulted in significant increases in all measures of genital blood flow. Furthermore, although older women had a lower baseline genital blood flow, there were no differences in genital blood flow after stimulation between younger and older women. In a subsequent study, Berman et al. [15] used the same methods to assess the therapeutic efficacy of sildenafil in 48 women with complaints of sexual dysfunction. Ultrasound measurements were taken at baseline and then 1 week later, after administration of 100 mg sildenafil. They were able to show a significant increase in all genital blood flow parameters as a result of stimulation and sildenafil.

The use of radiologic imaging in the diagnosis of male ED has decreased dramatically as a result of the successful introduction of the phosphodiesterase inhibitors and the recognition that surgical correction of penile vascular disease has poor outcomes. However, there are still some imaging techniques that are used in specific populations. The use of duplex Doppler ultrasonography in the assessment of the penile vasculature was first described in 1985 [16]. In this study, 2 normal healthy controls and 21 men with suspected vasculogenic impotence were recruited to undergo ultrasound assessment. They were first scanned in the flaccid state and then erections were induced via injection of papaverine into the corpus cavernosum. Measurements and Dopplers were repeated at 1, 3 and 5 min after injection. They were able to visualize the penile vasculature as well as calculate blood flow rates in the deep and dorsal penile arteries, indicating the diagnostic potential of duplex Doppler ultrasound for arterial vasculogenic impotence.

Using this same methodology, another group designed a study to see if the same imaging technique could be used to assess venous leakage – another possible mechanism for ED [17]. They recruited 45 patients and divided them into 5 groups: (1) psychogenic, (2) mild to moderate arterial insufficiency, (3) severe arterial insufficiency, (4) venous incompetence and (5) venous incompetence with mild to moderate arterial insufficiency. While they were able to detect significant dorsal venous leaks, they were not readily able to discern cavernosal venous leaks.

Color Doppler ultrasound uses standard ultrasound methods to produce a picture of a blood vessel. In addition, a computer converts the Doppler sounds into colors that are overlaid on the image of the blood vessel and that represent the speed and direction of blood flow through the vessel. Khalifé et al. [18] showed that clitoral blood flow in women who are not sexually aroused could be reliably assessed using this modality. In that study, they found high positive correlations between examiners for measurement of maximum velocity, resistance, and pulsatility. However, subsequent studies have shown that measurement of clitoral blood flow using this method has not been successful in differentiating sexual arousal from a humor control condition. Furthermore, there were no significant correlations between clitoral blood flow measures and subjective sexual arousal [19]. One study has, however, demonstrated a positive correlation between labial and clitoral blood flow and subjective arousal in women with type I diabetes who were treated with sildenafil [20].

More recently, color ultrasound has been the preferred method of evaluating ED, due to its superior ability to visualize the cavernosal arteries and the events occurring during erection. In a study of 10 healthy volunteers and 39 men with abnormal erectile function, Schwartz et al. [21] were able to use color Doppler ultrasound to discern between normal controls and men with various types of ED using the resultant waveform.

The advantages of ultrasound are that it is a quick, relatively easy, and noninvasive technique that provides a continuous, real-time, anatomic assessment (blood flow and volumetric). It can also assess changes in genital and vascular diameter associated with sexual stimulation [22]. The movement artifacts can be minimized. Most importantly, it provides measurements in absolute units that can be used for comparisons in research studies. It has also proven useful in determining the presence of genital calcifications secondary to trauma, which may cause sexual dysfunction [23]. Disadvantages include the need for the examiner to be in the room and a lack of standardization in terms of proper technique (i.e. placement of the probe). Vasoactive agents may be needed to facilitate smooth muscle relaxation to yield optimal vascular responses. The agents used to induce erection, such as papaverine, may cause potentially serious side effects in susceptible individuals. In men, significant anxiety can yield erroneous result, due to sympathetic outflow that results in vasoconstriction. Analysis of data requires experienced interpretation. So far, normative data in women have not been established, and low values do not necessarily correlate with sexual dysfunction. Though 'normative' data have been published for men, caution is still needed when confronted with intermediate values, which may result from intraobserver variation and varying definitions of endpoints.

Laser Doppler Perfusion Imaging

LDPI is a noninvasive method of measuring superficial skin microcirculatory blood flow. This modality can detect flow in capillaries as small as 11 μm and as deep as 2 mm below the skin surface. Sarrel used this technique to measure vaginal blood flow in postmenopausal women receiving estrogen versus estrogen-androgen treatment [24]. There were no significant differences in blood flow between the two groups. Laser Doppler flowmetry was also used to assess vaginal blood flow in 8 healthy women undergoing benign hysterectomy [25]. There were no significant differences found in blood flow before and after the procedure. The authors concluded that this method is an objective, reproducible measure of vaginal blood flow.

It has recently been used to measure vulvar blood flow changes during sexual arousal [26]. In this study, an LDPI scan was performed before and after reading a chapter of erotic fiction. The percentage change in flux was noted to significantly increase at the clitoris, labia, and posterior fourchette. An advantage of this method is that it is noninvasive, requiring minimal genital contact. It is reproducible and easy to perform. However, it is subject to movement artifact and the scans have to be performed in a dark environment that may preclude simultaneous measurement of other parameters. It also requires that the technician be present to hold the probe during the experiment, and is operator dependent. Furthermore, it cannot measure absolute perfusion and the flow is expressed in arbitrary laser Doppler flow units. Though this method is an easy way to assess vaginal blood flow, subsequent studies will be needed to determine its specificity, validity, and correlation with subjective measures of sexual function. We are not aware of use of LDPI for the assessment of sexual function or dysfunction in men.

Thermography

Thermography is a procedure in which a heat-sensing infrared camera is used to record the surface heat produced by different parts of the body. Essentially, increased vascularity can cause temperature changes, which may show up on a thermogram as in the case of many cancers. In fact, the first medical use of thermography was to aid in the diagnosis of breast cancer in the 1950s.

In the 1980s, Seeley et al. [27] were the first to apply the use of thermography to the measurement of sexual response. They based their studies on the premise that vasocongestion and myotonia are associated with increased temperature; thus, photographs of these heat patterns could quantify blood flow rate and transfer of heat in the genital tissues.

In their preliminary study, they assessed one male and one female, who were asked to masturbate to orgasm. Thermographic photos were taken of the subjects during initial masturbation, prior to orgasm, at the time of orgasm, and then after orgasm. Using these photos, a quantitative temperature profile was created. They found that there was a progressive increase in genital vasocongestion (with temperature increases up to above 3 degrees) during excitement and orgasm. During these phases, they also noted surface cooling of the abdomen.

In a second study by the same group, they sought to provide convergent validity for thermography, using the same methods with a larger group of subjects [28]. They recruited 37 women and 32 men, and randomly assigned them to 1 of 3 conditions: sexually arousing (which involved reading an excerpt from a sexually arousing story), emotionally arousing (which involved reading a passage from a fear/anger story) and a control group, where the subject stood there for the amount of time required to finish either story. A baseline thermograph was taken and another thermograph was taken after the study condition. Subjects were then asked to complete a scale of their reported sexual arousal. The authors found that subjects in the sexually arousing condition showed a significant increase in genital vasocongestion, while the other groups revealed a decrease. They also noted that genital vasocongestion significantly correlated with self-report of sexual arousal.

These findings stirred up interest in measuring extragenital areas, based on the notion that sexual response is not exclusive to only genital regions. Abramson et al. [29] used thermography to evaluate the pectoral region during sexual response. They studied three couples who attended two sessions: one in which they masturbated to orgasm and the other which served as a control session. The thermographic camera was focused on the pectoral region. They found that there was asymmetric vasocongestion in the right pectoral region and axilla for men and women and attributed this to the anatomy of the lymphatic system.

For many years, the work of Seeley and Abramson was abandoned, however, thermography may be experiencing somewhat of a renaissance. The availability of better technology and better cameras has renewed interest in the use of thermography in the measurement of sexual arousal. In 2007, Kukkonen et al. [30] published a study using thermography to assess sexual arousal in men and women. They recruited 28 men and 30 women to view a neutral film clip. After this clip, the subjects were randomly assigned to view one of three other video conditions: neutral, humor, or sexually explicit. During the viewings, genital and thigh temperatures were continuously recorded using a TSA ImagIR camera. Subjective measures of sexual arousal, humor, and relaxation were assessed prior to showing the baseline video and following each film. The authors found that both men and women viewing the sexually arousing video had significantly greater genital temperature than those in the humor or neutral conditions. Furthermore, men and women in the erotic condition did not differ from each other in time to peak genital temperature and genital temperature was significantly and highly correlated with subjective ratings of sexual arousal. While they showed that thermography can be used to differentiate sexual arousal from humor and neutral conditions, this study also stressed the similarities between men and women in terms of time to arousal and their subjective ratings of sexual arousal.

While promising, thermography has a set of unique advantages and limitations. What makes it particularly attractive is that it is noninvasive and can be used in both males and females. Furthermore, it bypasses individual anatomic variation, yields a body composite and shows a correlation with self-report measures of sexual arousal. However, it is very expensive, requiring highly specialized equipment and personnel knowledgeable on the use of the thermographic camera. From a methodological standpoint, there are concerns that use of the camera may affect arousal and that ambient temperature may affect the data. Finally, there is no standardized way to analyze the data.

Dynamic MRI

Dynamic MRI involves the acquisition of serial images before, during and after the injection of an MR contrast agent. Using this process, the functionality of a particular organ can be assessed. Deliganis et al. [31] used MRI with a contrast agent (MS-325, a gadolinium chelate) to monitor sexual response in 12 healthy sexually functional women. A baseline image was obtained and then MS-325 was administered. The subjects then viewed neutral and erotic video segments and images were taken every 3 min over a 45-min period. After watching the sexually oriented video clips, the MRI images showed strong contrast enhancement of the external genitalia and clitoris, with a significant increase in clitoral size. All women reported feeling sexually aroused. As part of this study, the investigators also calculated relative blood-flow and found that there were no difference in the change of blood flow between pre- and postmenopausal women. Subsequently, Suh et al. [32] described detailed female anatomy and anatomic changes in 12 healthy premenopausal and 9 healthy postmenopausal women using dynamic MRI with the same contrast agent. They found that the vagina was well visualized in premenopausal subjects but that there were not distinguishable mucosal rugae or clearly separate layers in postmenopausal subjects. Furthermore, postmenopausal subjects were also observed to have smaller labia minora width, vestibular bulb width, vaginal width and wall thickness, and cervical diameter. This was the first study to describe detailed female genital anatomy using MRI. The same group then used contrast-enhanced MRI to assess the anatomy of 11 healthy premenopausal women and 8 healthy menopausal women during sexual arousal [33]. Images of the pelvis were taken at baseline and following the viewing of erotic film clips. Measurements of selected genital structures were taken at baseline and after arousal. They found that the vestibular bulb, labia minora and clitoris showed increased enhancement in pre- and postmenopausal subjects while there were no significant changes in the enhancement or size of the labia majora, urethra, cervix, or rectum. There was significant enhancement of the vagina in only the premenopausal subjects.

Once it was established that contrast-enhanced MRI could effectively assess female genital anatomy, there were efforts to develop imaging technique that did not require the use of contrast. Maravilla et al. [34] evaluated the use of dynamic noncontrast MRI and T_2-weighted images of female genitalia for quantitative evaluation of female sexual arousal response. In this study, 8 women attended two separate MRI sessions where they were shown sexually oriented video clips. MRI images were taken at 3-min intervals over 45 min. All women reported feeling sexually aroused. Images were analyzed for clitoral volume and percent change in clitoral volume. The investigators found excellent intrasubject reproducibility between sessions as well as with their prior noncontrast studies.

Yang et al. [35] performed a histological study with MRI to assess vulvar tissues. The histologic specimens consisted of 7 cadaveric vulvectomy samples; in addition, 1 healthy premenopausal and 1 healthy postmenopausal woman with normal sexual functioning was recruited to undergo contrast-enhanced MRI with MS-325. Baseline images were taken. They were shown erotic film clips as described by previous protocols and MRI images were taken. From the cadaveric vulvectomy specimens, there were noted to be 5 vascular compartments, each of which consisted of erectile or nonerectile specialized genital tissue. Correlation with MRI revealed that the erectile tissues (corpus cavernosum of the clitoris and the bulbs) showed the greatest change in enhancement on MRI.

In men, MRI has been used to delineate male genital structures in normal men and men with various penile conditions. With regard to the workup of ED, Hricak et al. [36] used MRI to observe penile anatomy in 4 subjects with vasculogenic impotence. Images were taken in the flaccid state and 5 min after the injection of papaverine. In those subjects, the corpus spongiosum showed no changes in size or signal intensity from the flaccid to erect state; however, the corpus cavernosum was noted to increase in size and signal intensity.

The development of a noninvasive angiographic method was reported by Stehling et al. [37], who used contrast-enhanced magnetic resonance angiography (MRA) to provide a three-dimensional picture of the pelvic vasculature in men. Eleven patients with ED were recruited to undergo MRA. Films were taken in the flaccid state and then the corpus cavernosum was injected with 20 μm of prostaglandin E. In addition, a contrast agent was injected. Using this technique, they were able to see the small vessels of the penis that were not readily identifiable using previous methods.

Subsequently, MRI has been used to assess venous leakage in patients with ED. In one study, 28 patients with venooclusive ED were evaluated with MRI and enhancement by intracavernous injection of paramagnetic contrast agent [38]. Erection was induced using 40 mg of papaverine. They found that MRI confirmed the diagnosis in all 28 patients and provided additional information such as venous leakage type and location which could not be documented by more conventional methods (such as dynamic infusion cavernosometry and cavernosography). They suggested that this technique could be useful in the planning of surgical treatment and may become part of the clinical algorithm for diagnosis in certain subsets of men with ED.

The advantages of using MRI to study female and male sexual response include its excellent visualization of anatomic detail, noninvasiveness, and reproducibility.

Newer techniques do not require use of contrast, which limits the risk to patient, decreases expense, and eliminates the need to establish vascular access. Disadvantages include high costs, time requirement, and machine unavailability. Subjects also must be appropriate candidates for MRI (no metallic substances in/on the body) and be able to remain stationary during the testing session. Use of MRA in males allows for rapid and superior visualization of small vessels, although patency of these small vessels cannot be accurately confirmed. In addition, MRA is less invasive and cheaper than angiography, the gold standard.

Neuroimaging

One of the most exciting developments in the study of sexual function is the use of neuroimaging techniques to help clarify the neural substrates of human sexual behavior. Prior to the availability of this technology, such information could only be gained by animal studies or human research involving neurosurgical lesions. However, using imaging modalities such as single-photon emission computed tomography (SPECT), positron emission tomography (PET) and fMRI, we can now study functioning systems in healthy human brains.

Single-Photon Emission Computed Tomography

The first attempts to employ neuroimaging to look at sexual function were made by Tiihonen et al. [39] in 1994 using SPECT. SPECT uses gamma ray-emitting radioisotopes and a gamma camera to record data that a computer uses to construct two- or three-dimensional images of active brain regions. It requires use of a radioactive tracer that is rapidly taken up by the brain, but does not redistribute. This group sought to observe cerebral activation by sexual stimulation during orgasm. To do this, they measured cerebral blood flow (CBF) in 8 healthy young males using Tc-HMPAO (a gamma-emitting radionuclide imaging agent) and high-resolution SPECT. They found that 4/8 of the subjects had a significant increase in CBF in right prefrontal lobe; however, other areas of the brain were unchanged or decreased. It was concluded that this area was important for emotional responses concerning human male sexuality.

One of the benefits of SPECT is the rapid uptake of radiotracer; thus, the resultant image represents the cerebral state at the time of injection. In addition, the radiotracers used have longer half-lives than those used in other modalities, such as PET, making them easier to produce and therefore, more readily available. However, the resolution achieved with SPECT is not as clear as other imaging.

Positron Emission Tomography

PET neuroimaging is based on the assumption that areas of high radioactivity are associated with brain activity. What is actually measured indirectly is the flow of blood to different parts of the brain, and this has been measured using the tracer oxygen-15. It provides a computerized image of the metabolic activity of the cerebral tissues to localize functional response. Most PET studies of sexual arousal have been performed in men.

Stoléru et al. [40] were the first to use PET to study visually evoked sexual arousal in men. Eight healthy young men were studied in 3 different conditions; they were shown silent video clips of three types: sexually arousing, neutral and humorous. They found a pattern of increased rCBF in the inferior temporal cortex, a visual association area, the right insula and right inferior frontal cortex, which are two paralimbic areas relating highly processed sensory information with motivational states, and the left anterior cingulate cortex, another paralimbic area known to control autonomic and neuroendocrine functions. They concluded that PET had the ability to identify brain regions associated with sexual arousal in men.

Rauch et al. [41] used PET in a paradigm where 8 healthy young men had to recall and imagine an event (using prepared scripts) associated either with sexual arousal or 'competitive arousal' compared with a neutral condition. They reported that both arousal conditions were characterized by increased activation within the anterior cingulated and anterior temporal cortex and the ventral globus pallidus. However, the sexually arousing paradigm specifically resulted in the activation of the brain stem and in the left claustrum.

Redouté et al. [42], building upon the findings of Stoléru, recruited 9 healthy right-handed heterosexual men and imaged them using PET while they were exposed to erotic video clips and photographs of graded intensity. This study confirmed the findings of the Stoléru study. In addition, they were able to note activation in additional areas including the claustrum, the putamens, thalami, hypothalamus, nucleus accumbens, central sulcus and parietal lobules due to the higher resolution achieved by a better whole-brain PET scanner. This study utilized a sample of older subjects, which made it more applicable to the general population. It suggested that sexual arousal in males requires functional changes in multiple brain regions.

In addition to these seminal studies, additional studies of sexual arousal using PET in men have been done. In 2001, Bocher et al. [43] utilized PET in 10 young healthy males watching erotic film clips and found that sexual arousal was mainly associated with activation of bilateral, predominantly right, inferoposterior extrastriate cortices, of the right inferolateral prefrontal cortex and of the midbrain. PET has also been explored as a potential diagnostic modality to identify men with hypoactive sexual desire disorder (HSDD) [44]. Seven male patients with HSDD and 8 healthy men were compared on their regional CBF (rCBF) responses to visual sexual stimuli of graded intensity. While the medial orbitofrontal cortex showed a deactivation in response to sexual stimuli in control subjects, HSDD patients had an abnormally maintained activity of this region, which has been implicated in the inhibitory control of motivated behavior. Redouté et al. [45] used PET to determine the difference in cerebral activation in 9 hypogonadal males versus 8 healthy males. Activation was higher in controls than in untreated hypogonadal patients in the right orbitofrontal cortex, insula and claustrum; notably, activation in these areas increased when the hypogonadal men were treated with testosterone.

In addition to diagnostic utility, researchers were interested in learning about neuroanatomic correlates that are activated over the course of the sexual cycle. Georgiadis and Holstege [46] used PET to measure cerebral activation during various stages of sexual performance in men. Compared to a passive resting condition (without penile erection), sexual stimulation of the penis increased rCBF in an area of the right hemisphere encompassing the posterior insula and adjacent posterior part of the secondary somatosensory cortex and decreased rCBF in the right amygdala. No activation was observed in either the thalamus, genital part of primary somatosensory cortex, or hypothalamus. They concluded that the absence of activation in the hypothalamus indicates that it is more important for the onset of sexual arousal than for the resulting sexual performance and that deactivation of the amygdala during sexual stimulation of the penis corresponds with a decrease of vigilance during sexual performance. In another study, Miyagawa et al. [47] analyzed rCBF of 6 healthy volunteers during the plateau phase (maintenance of penile erection) induced by erotic videos and compared the results with those of the excitation phase. During the plateau phase, primary subcortical activation was noted in the right ventral putamen, indicating motivational factors in the sexual response via the limbic reward circuit. A significant increase in rCBF in the left hypothalamus was also observed during the plateau phase. The right anterior cingulate and left insula were specifically activated during the excitation phase but not during the plateau phase. These results indicate a significant role of the ventral putamen and the hypothalamus in the plateau phase and confirm that paralimbic and limbic components of the human brain differentially coordinate the sexual response in a psychosexual phase-dependent manner.

Very few studies using PET to assess sexual function and arousal in women exist. Whipple and Komisaruk [48] performed a PET-MRI study on 2 women with complete spinal cord injury and 1 woman with no injuries. They found that cervical self-stimulation increased activity in the region of the nucleus of the solitary tract, which is the brainstem nucleus to which the vagus nerves project, suggesting that the vagus nerves can convey genital sensory input directly to the brain in women, completely bypassing SCI at any level.

Georgiadis et al. [49] used PET to measure rCBF in 12 healthy women during rest, clitoral-induced orgasm, sexual clitoral stimulation and imitation of orgasm. They found that during sexual stimulation, there was activation of the left secondary and right dorsal primary somatosensory cortex, while during orgasm there were decreases in the neocortex – especially the left lateral orbitofrontal cortex, inferior temporal gyrus, and anterior temporal pole. They postulated that decreases in the left lateral orbitofrontal cortex signifies behavioral disinhibition during orgasm and that deactivation of the temporal lobe is directly related to high sexual arousal.

The advantage of PET is that it permits functional assessment and is less subject to movement artifacts. However, disadvantages of this modality are that it is invasive, and requires the use of radiolabeled compounds. It is relatively expensive and the rapid decay of radioactivity limits evaluation to short tasks. Subject individuality makes comparisons between subjects difficult. Furthermore, its resolution is inferior to that of fMRI, limiting its clinical use.

Functional MRI

Functional MRI involves obtaining three-dimensional images of the brain based on changes in blood flow and that can be correlated with brain functions. Recently, there have been many studies utilizing this technique to study sexual response in men and women. This review is not meant to be exhaustive, but rather highlight a few notable studies.

One of the earliest reports of the use of fMRI for the study of sexual response was by Risinger et al. [50], who reported on the use of fMRI to study sexual arousal in 5 males. The subjects were shown static images while undergoing MRI. It was found that the bilateral inferior temporal and middle occipital brain regions were activated in response to these static sexual images. While this study yielded new information, it had significant limitations, including a small sample size and use of static images instead of video clips.

In 2001, Beauregard et al. [51] used fMRI to study brain activation in normal male subjects while they either responded in a normal manner to erotic film excerpts or voluntarily attempted to inhibit the sexual arousal induced by viewing erotic stimuli. They found that sexual arousal was associated with activation in limbic and paralimbic structures, including the right amygdala, right anterior temporal pole, and hypothalamus. However, inhibition of sexual arousal was associated with activation of the right superior frontal gyrus and right anterior cingulate gyrus and no activation was found in limbic areas. The authors concluded that 'emotional self-regulation is normally implemented by a neural circuit comprising various prefrontal regions and subcortical limbic structures'.

Park et al. [52] evaluated the cerebral centers of penile erection using blood-oxygen level-dependent fMRI (BOLD-functional MRI). fMRI was performed on 12 normal male volunteers and two hypogonadal impotent patients.Visual stimulation was achieved using a combined erotic and nonerotic film to identify and quantify the activated brain regions associated with sexual response. Subjective sexual arousal and penile erection responses were also assessed. The occipital cortex was activated by both the erotic and nonerotic film, but the erotic film gave 150–200% stronger activation. Seven of the 12 healthy subjects showed significant activation in the areas of inferior frontal lobe, cingulate gyrus, insula gyrus, corpus callosum, thalamus, caudate nucleus, globus pallidus, and inferior temporal lobe by erotic stimulation. In the hypogonadal patients, brain activation in response to the erotic film decreased compared to normal volunteers; however, it was restored by testosterone supplementation.

Arnow et al. [53] used fMRI to study sexual arousal in a group of young, healthy, heterosexual males. Each subject was exposed to two sequences of video material consisting of explicitly erotic, relaxing, and sports segments. Penile turgidity was also measured. Strong activations specifically associated with penile turgidity were observed in the right subinsular region including the claustrum, left caudate and putamen, right middle occipital/middle temporal gyri, bilateral cingulate gyrus and right sensorimotor and premotor regions. Smaller, but significant activation was observed in the right hypothalamus.

Functional MRI studies of sexual arousal have also been performed in women. Park et al. [54] used functional MRI to identify and quantify brain regions associated with visually evoked sexual arousal in women. They found that the inferior frontal lobe, cingulate gyrus, insula gyrus, corpus callosum, thalamus, caudate nucleus, globus pallidus and inferior temporal lobe were significantly activated. Another study used functional MRI to investigate the differences in brain activity in response to sexually oriented visual stimuli between men and women [55]. It was found that subjective ratings of sexual arousal were significantly greater in men than in women. Though significant activation of the medial prefrontal cortex, orbital frontal cortex, anterior cingulate cortex, insular cortex, occipitotemporal cortex, amygdala and ventral striatum occurred in both sexes, males showed a significant activation in the thalamus and hypothalamus while females did not. Furthermore, a positive correlation between subjective arousal and the magnitude of hypothalamic activation in men was made but this correlation was not made in women. Using fMRI, it has also been shown that the activated brain center associated with visually evoked sexual arousal showed qualitative and quantitative differences between premenopausal and menopausal women [56]. Another study found that women in the mid-luteal phase exhibited differences in cerebral activation than women outside the luteal phase; however, gender differences with women in both phases remained the same [57]. A recent study using fMRI showed that administration of estradiol and testosterone to surgically menopausal women resulted in increased brain activation and enhanced limbic response to erotic visual stimulation, compared to baseline [58].

An advantage of using fMRI is that it is a safe, noninvasive means by which to examine sexual arousal in terms of the central nervous system. It provides superior visualization of neural tissue. However, it is expensive, time-consuming, and limited in its ability to measure absolute neural activity. As with any MRI study, subjects must be appropriate candidates. Standardization protocols need to be developed to determine what strength of scanner should be used. Furthermore, more studies are needed to validate this method before it can be used for clinical research studies.

Advantages and Limitations of Imaging

The use of imaging in the study of male and female sexual function and dysfunction has certainly contributed to our knowledge of these processes. Moreover, certain imaging modalities have allowed for comparison between the sexes, which has been difficult to achieve using psychophysiologic methods.

However, there are significant limitations inherent to the use of imaging. First and foremost, sexual response is a complex entity that has multiple components; imaging will not give us a complete understanding of this process. In addition, methodology and paradigm design – especially in the area of neuroimaging – can really influence findings. For example, there is a lack of standardization of erotic stimuli used to induce sexual arousal, which may significantly affect the magnitude of sexual response elicited. Woodard et al. [59] attempted to address this issue by determining what type of erotic video clips optimize sexual response in women, though physiologic parameters were not measured in that study. Furthermore, individual subject differences as well as the arduous task of trying to isolate sexual response are additional methodological challenges. All imaging modalities require the use of costly machinery and subjects must be studied in 'unnatural' environments, which may be inhibitory to sexual response. All imaging is subject to interpretation and standardization in this area will be needed to be able to compare findings between studies. While some imaging modalities appear to show correlations between subjective and physiologic arousal, it remains to be seen whether these continue to hold true for others – particularly in women.

Conclusions

Imaging can provide insight into the anatomy, physiology, and functional neuroanatomy of male and female sexual function and dysfunction. In addition to exploratory endeavors, it has the potential to aid in diagnosis and evaluate therapeutic efficacy. While promising, more research is needed to optimize its use in the field of sexology.

References

1 Clark K, Pedretti O: The drawings of Leonardo da Vinci in the collection of Her Majesty the Queen at Windsor Castle. London, Phaidon, 1968.

2 Dickinson RL: Human Sex Anatomy, A topographical hand atlas (2nd ed.). London, Braillier, Tindall and Cox, 1949.

3 Masters WH, Johnson VE: Human sexual response. Boston, Little, Brown, 1966.

4 Barnhart KT, Pretorius ES, Stolpen A, Malamud D: Distribution of topical medication in the human vagina as imaged by MRI. Fertil Steril 2001;76: 189–195.

5 Riley AJ, Lees W, Riley EJ: An ultrasound study of human coitus; in Bezemer W, Cohen-Kettenis P, Slob K, Van Son-Schoones N (eds): Sex Matters. Amsterdam, Elsevier, 1992, pp 29–36.

6 Deng J, Hall-Craggs MA, Pellerin D, Linney AD, Lees WR, Rodeck CH, Todd-Pokropek A: Real-time three-dimensional ultrasound visualization of erection and artificial coitus. Int J Androl 2006;29: 374–379.

7 Schultz WW, van Andel P, Sabelis I, Mooyaart E: Magnetic resonance imaging of male and female genitals during coitus and female sexual arousal. BMJ 1999;319:1596–1600.

8 Faix A, Lapray JF, Courtieu C, Maubon A, Lanfrey K: Magnetic resonance imaging of sexual intercourse: initial experience. J Sex Marital Ther 2001;27: 475–482.
9 Faix A, Lapray JF, Callede O, Maubon A, Lanfrey K: Magnetic resonance imaging (MRI) of sexual intercourse: second experience in missionary position and initial experience in posterior position. J Sex Marital Ther 2002;28(suppl 1):63–76.
10 Goldstein I, De EJB, Johnson JA: Persistent sexual arousal syndrome and clitoral priapism; in Goldstein I, Meston CM, Davis SR, Traish AM (eds): Women's Sexual Function and Dysfunction: Study, Diagnosis and Treatment. London, Taylor and Francis, 1995, pp 674–688.
11 Lavoisier P, Aloui R, Schmidt MH, Watrelot A: Clitoral blood flow increases following vaginal pressure stimulation. Arch Sex Behav 1995;24:37–45.
12 Becher EF, Bechara A, Casabe A: Clitoral hemodynamic changes after a topical application of alprostadil. J Sex Marital Ther 2001;27:405–410.
13 Bechara A, Bertolino MV, Casabé A, Munarriz R, Goldstein I, Morin A, Secin F, Literat B, Pesaresi M, Fredotovich N: Duplex Doppler ultrasound assessment of clitoral hemodynamics after topical administration of alprostadil in women with arousal and orgasmic disorders. J Sex Marital Ther 2003;29 (suppl):1–10.
14 Berman JR, Berman LA, Werbin TJ, Flaherty EE, Leahy NM, Goldstein I: Clinical evaluation of female sexual function: effects of age and estrogen status on subjective and physiologic sexual responses. Int J Impot Res 1999;11:S31–S38.
15 Berman JR, Berman LA, Lin H, Flaherty E, Lahey N, Goldstein I, Cantey-Kiser J: Effect of Sildenafil on subjective and physiologic parameters of the female sexual response in women with sexual arousal disorder. J Sex Marital Ther 2001;27:411–420.
16 Lue TF, Hricak H, Marich KW, Tanagho EA: Vasculogenic impotence evaluated by high-resolution ultrasonography and pulsed Doppler spectrum analysis. Radiology 1985;155:777–781.
17 Benson CB, Vickers MA: Sexual impotence caused by vascular disease: diagnosis with duplex sonography. AJR Am J Roentgenol 1989;153:1149–1153.
18 Khalifé S, Binik YM, Cohen DR, Amsel R: Evaluation of clitoral blood flow by color Doppler ultrasonography. J Sex Marital Ther 2000;32:243–251.
19 Kukkonen TM, Paterson L, Binik YM, Amsel R, Bouvier F, Khalife S: Convergent and discriminant validity of clitoral color Doppler ultrasonography as a measure of female sexual arousal. J Sex Marital Ther 2006;32:281–287.
20 Caruso S, Rugolo S, Agnello C, Intelisano G, Di Mari L, Cianci A: Sildenafil improves sexual functioning in premenopausal women with type 1 diabetes who are affected by sexual arousal disorder: a double-blind, crossover, placebo-controlled pilot study. Fertil Steril 2006;85:1496–1501.
21 Schwartz AN, Lowe M, Berger RE, Wang KY, Mack LA, Richardson ML: Assessment of normal and abnormal erectile function: color Doppler flow sonography versus conventional techniques. Radiology 1991;180:105–109.
22 Nader SG, Maitland SR, Munarriz R, Goldstein I: Blood flow: duplex Doppler ultrasound; in Goldstein I, Meston CM, Davis SR, Traish AM (eds): Women's Sexual Function and Dysfunction: Study, Diagnosis and Treatment. London, Taylor and Francis, 1995, pp 383–390.
23 Frauscher F, Klauser A, Stenzl A, Helweg G, Amort B, zur Nedden D: US findings in the scrotum of extreme mountain bikers. Radiology 2001;219:427–431.
24 Sarrel PM: Ovarian hormones and vaginal blood flow: using laser Doppler velocimetry to measure effects in a clinical trial of post-menopausal women. Int J Impot Res 1998;10:S91–S93.
25 Richman SM, Sarrel PM: Vaginal laser Doppler flowmetry pre- and posthysterectomy. J Sex Marital Ther 2004;30:43–47.
26 Styles SJ, Maclean AB, Reid WM, Sultana SR: Laser Doppler perfusion imaging: a method for measuring female sexual response. BJOG 2006;113:599–601.
27 Seeley TT, Abramson PR, Perry LB, Rothblatt AB, Seeley DM: Thermographic measurement of sexual arousal: a methodological note. Arch Sex Behav 1980; 9:77–85.
28 Abramson PR, Perry LB, Seeley TT, Seeley DM, Rothblatt AB: Thermographic measurement of sexual arousal: a discriminant validity analysis. Arch Sex Behav 1981;10:171–176.
29 Abramson PR, Pearsall EH: Pectoral changes during the sexual response cycle: a thermographic analysis. Arch Sex Behav 1983;12:357–368.
30 Kukkonen TM, Binik YM, Amsel R, Carrier S: Thermography as a physiological measure of sexual arousal in both men and women. J Sex Med 2007;4: 93–105.
31 Deliganis AV, Maravilla KR, Heiman JR, Carter WO, Garland PA, Peterson BT, Hackbert L, Cao Y, Weisskoff RM: Female genitalia: dynamic MR imaging with use of MS-325-initial experiences evaluating female sexual response. Radiology 2002; 225:791–799.
32 Suh DD, Yang CC, Cao Y, Garland PA, Maravilla KR: Magnetic resonance imaging anatomy of the female genitalia in premenopausal and postmenopausal women. J Urol 2003;170:138–144.

33 Suh DD, Yang CC, Cao Y, Heiman JR, Garland PA, Maravilla KR: MRI of female genital and pelvic organs during sexual arousal. J Psychosom Obstet Gynaecol 2004;2:153–162.

34 Maravilla KR, Cao Y, Heiman JR, Yang C, Garland PA, Peterson BT, Carter WO: Noncontrast dynamic magnetic resonance imaging for quantitative assessment of female sexual arousal. J Urol 2005;173:162–166.

35 Yang CC, Cold CJ, Yilmaz U, Maravilla KR: Sexually responsive vascular tissue of the vulva. BJU Int 2006;97:766–772.

36 Hricak H, Marotti M, Gilbert TJ, Lue TF, Wetzel LH, McAninch JW, Tanagho EA: Normal penile anatomy and abnormal penile conditions: evaluation with MR imaging. Radiology 1988;169:683–690.

37 Stehling MK, Liu L, Laub G, Fleischmann K, Rohde U: Gadolinium-enhanced magnetic resonance angiography of the pelvis in patients with erectile impotence. MAGMA 1997;5:247–254.

38 Kurbatov DG, Kuznetsky YY, Kitaev SV, Brusensky VA: Magnetic resonance imaging as a potential tool for objective visualization of venous leakage in patients with veno-occlusive erectile dysfunction. Int J Impot Res 2007; in press.

39 Tiihonen J, Kuikka J, Kupila J, Partanen K, Vainio P, Airaksinen J, Eronen M, Hallikainen T, Paanila J, Kinnunen I: Increase in cerebral blood flow of right prefrontal cortex in man during orgasm. Neurosci Lett 1994;170:241–243.

40 Stoléru S, Grégoire MC, Gérard D, Decety J, Lafarge E, Cinotti L, Lavenne F, Le Bars D, Vernet-Maury E, Rada H, Collet C, Mazoyer B, Forest MG, Magnin F, Spira A, Comar D: Neuroanatomical correlates of visually evoked sexual arousal in human males. Arch Sex Behav 1999;28:1–21.

41 Rauch SL, Shin LM, Dougherty DD, Alpert NM, Orr SP, Lasko M, Macklin ML, Fischman AJ, Pitman RK: Neural activation during sexual and competitive arousal in healthy men. Psychiatry Res 1999;91:1–10.

42 Redouté J, Stoléru S, Grégoire MC, Costes N, Cinotti L, Lavenne F, Le Bars D, Forest MG, Pujol JF: Brain processing of visual sexual stimuli in human males. Hum Brain Mapp 2000;11:162–177.

43 Bocher M, Chisin R, Parag Y, Freedman N, Meir Weil Y, Lester H, Mishani E, Bonne O: Cerebral activation associated with sexual arousal in response to a pornographic clip: A 15O-H2O PET study in heterosexual men. Neuroimage 2001;14:105–117.

44 Stoléru S, Redouté J, Costes N, Lavenne F, Bars DL, Dechaud H, Forest MG, Pugeat M, Cinotti L, Pujol JF: Brain processing of visual sexual stimuli in men with hypoactive sexual desire disorder. Psychiatry Res 2003;124:67–86.

45 Redouté J, Stoléru S, Pugeat M, Costes N, Lavenne F, Le Bars D, Dechaud H, Cinotti L, Pujol JF: Brain processing of visual sexual stimuli in treated and untreated hypogonadal patients. Psychoneuroendocrinology 2005;30:461–482.

46 Georgiadis JR, Holstege G: Human brain activation during sexual stimulation of the penis. J Comp Neurol 2005;493:33–38.

47 Miyagawa Y, Tsujimura A, Fujita K, Matsuoka Y, Takahashi T, Takao T, Takada S, Matsumiya K, Osaki Y, Takasawa M, Oku N, Hatazawa J, Kaneko S, Okuyama A: Differential brain processing of audiovisual sexual stimuli in men: comparative positron emission tomography study of the initiation and maintenance of penile erection during sexual arousal. Neuroimage 2007;36:830–842.

48 Whipple B, Komisaruk BR: Brain (PET) responses to vaginal-cervical self-stimulation in women with complete spinal cord injury: preliminary findings. J Sex Marital Ther 2002;28:79–86.

49 Georgiadis JR, Kortekaas R, Kuipers R, Nieuwenburg A, Pruim J, Reinders AA, Holstege G: Regional cerebral blood flow changes associated with clitorally induced orgasm in healthy women. Eur J Neurosci 2006;24:3305–3316.

50 Risinger RC, Garavan H, Kelley DJ, Ross TJ, Salmeron BJ, Stein EA: Valence vs. arousal: fRMI of emotional stimuli. Neuroimage 1999;9:s357.

51 Beauregard M, Lévesque J, Bourgouin P: Neural correlates of conscious self-regulation of emotion. J Neurosci 2001;21:RC165.

52 Park K, Seo JJ, Kang HK, Ryu SB, Kim HJ, Jeong GW: A new potential of blood oxygenation level dependent (BOLD) functional MRI for evaluating cerebral centers of penile erection. Int J Impot Res 2001;13:73–81.

53 Arnow BA, Desmond JE, Banner LL, Glover GH, Solomon A, Polan ML, Lue TF, Atlas SW: Brain activation and sexual arousal in healthy, heterosexual males. Brain 2002;125:1014–1023.

54 Park K, Kang, HK, Seo JJ, Kim HJ, Ryu SB, Jeong GW: Blood-oxygenation-level-dependent functional magnetic resonance imaging for evaluating cerebral regions of female sexual arousal response. Urology 2001;57:1189–1194.

55 Karama S, Lecours AR, Leroux JM, Bourgouin P, Beaudoin G, Joubert S, Beauregard M: Areas of brain activation in males and females during viewing of erotic film excerpts. Hum Brain Mapp 2002;16:1–13.

56 Jeong GW, Park K, Youn G, Kang HK, Kim HJ, Seo JJ, Ryu SB: Assessment of cerebrocortical regions associated with sexual arousal in premenopausal and menopausal women by using BOLD-based functional MRI. J Sex Med 2005;2:645–651.
57 Gizewski ER, Krause E, Karama S, Baars A, Senf W, Forsting M: There are differences in cerebral activation between females in distinct menstrual phases during viewing of erotic stimuli: a fMRI study. Exp Brain Res 2006;174:101–108.
58 Archer JS, Love-Geffen TE, Herbst-Damm KL, Swinney DA, Chang JR: Effect of estradiol and testosterone on brain-activation patterns in postmenopausal women. Menopause 2006;13:528–537.
59 Woodard TL, Collins K, Perez M, Balon R, Tancer ME, Kruger M, Moffat S, Diamond MP: What kind of erotic film clips should we use in female sex research? An exploratory study. J Sex Med 2008; 5:146–154.

Terri L. Woodard, MD
Wayne State University School of Medicine, Department of Obstetrics and Gynecology, Division of Reproductive Endocrinology and Infertility
3750 Woodward Avenue Suite 200D
Detroit, MI 48201 (USA)
Tel. +1 313 993 4525, Fax +1 313 993 4534, E-Mail twoodard@med.wayne.edu

Subject Index